Dirty

MW01290893

Lose Weight and Get in Great Shape Without Following Strict Ketogenic Rules

Thomas Rohmer

Disclaimer:

This guide has been created for informational and reference purposes only. The author, publisher, and any other affiliated parties cannot be held in any way accountable for any personal injuries or damage allegedly resulting from the information contained herein, or from any misuse of such guidance. Although strict measures have been taken to provide accurate information, the parties involved with the creation and publication of this guide take no responsibility for any issues that may arise from alleged discrepancies contained herein. It is strongly recommended that you consult a physician, personal trainer, and nutritionist prior to commencing this or any other workout or diet plan. This guide is not a substitute for professional personal guidance from a qualified medical professional. If you feel pain or discomfort at any point during exercises contained herein, cease the activity immediately and seek medical guidance.

Before You Begin:

Get the Latest Scoop on the Most Cutting Edge Info on Health & Fitness!

As thanks for picking up this book, I'd love to offer you the chance to maximize your results by getting exclusive info on health and fitness.

You'll be the first to know when I publish new books, and you'll receive exclusive content on health and fitness that I only share with people on my list.

Simply visit the link directly below and get started on the path to the healthiest version of yourself today!

https://rohmerfitness.lpages.co/kindle-sign-up/

Table of Contents

Introduction

Obesity is at an all-time high in America. This shouldn't be the case considering that we now have access to more information than we ever did before.

We have access to the latest information in nutrition, exercise, and supplementation, yet things only seem to be getting worse. The problem comes down to two main things.

The first is that we're being fed the wrong information. Yes, having access to a lot of information is great, assuming it's beneficial information. Sadly, this isn't the case most of the time, which is what keeps most of us stuck where we're at.

For example, a supplement company may promote things that aren't the full truth about their product so that they can increase sales. People may buy that supplement with the hope that they can achieve a certain result, when in reality, the supplement won't work. It wasn't the person's fault; they were just being told the wrong information, which is why he or she isn't getting the desired result.

Other times, the information might be good and factual but way too hard for the average individual to stick with. For example, some diet plans severely limit what foods you can and can't eat.

There may very well be a lot of good information that exists about that diet, but it could be too hard for the average individual to stick with for a prolonged period of time. If you quit on a diet, then you don't have any chance of success. A diet is only good as long as you can keep on doing it.

This is why it's so important to not only have the right information but also the right plan. You need both in order to succeed.

The right information with the wrong plan will cause you to quit, and the wrong information with the right plan will cause you to make mistakes that will hold you back.

That's why I plan to change things with this book. I'm going to give you the right information and the right plan in order to help you succeed. The plan we're going to use is the dirty ketogenic diet.

This is going to give us more flexibility than the regular keto diet, which will help make it a long-term sustainable diet. Additionally, you're also going to learn the correct way to do the dirty keto diet.

The reason why I say this is because it can be easy to approach the dirty keto diet with the wrong mentality. If you approach it thinking you can eat whatever you want as long as you're not eating carbs, then you have a long road ahead of you.

Yes, the dirty keto diet is awesome because it allows you to eat certain foods you normally wouldn't be able to on a standard keto diet, but you have to do it in the right way. That's what you're going to learn how to do in this book.

You're going to learn the proper way to do the dirty keto diet so that you can continue doing it for a long time to come. In fact, my goal is to make things to where it doesn't even feel like a diet.

The process needs to be as effortless as possible in order to get the best results. Don't get me wrong, sacrifices will have to be made; losing weight isn't a walk in the park. However, that doesn't mean we need to make things harder on ourselves for no good reason.

The dirty keto diet can help you reach your goal bodyweight and stay there for good. All that's left is to learn the necessary information, but before we get into that, would you please consider leaving a review for this book if you enjoy it? Even just a few words will help other people know if the book is right for them.

Many thanks in advance!

Chapter 1: What is the Standard Ketogenic Diet?

Before I get into the ins and outs of the dirty keto diet, it's important to first understand what the regular ketogenic diet is. The ketogenic diet is a high fat, moderate protein, and low-carb diet.

It was first recommended in the 1920's to help patients with epilepsy control their seizures. When people first hear about the ketogenic diet and how much fat you eat, they're usually alarmed.

This should come as no surprise since we've been told most of our lives that fat is bad for you. It can take a while to break through that mindset even after you've started the ketogenic diet.

In fact, when a lot of people first start a keto diet, they don't eat as much fat as they should! Again, a lot of this has to do with the lies we've been told about fats.

Now the point of the ketogenic diet is to get our bodies to use fat as fuel instead of carbohydrates. That's why the fat intake is so high on a ketogenic diet.

Our bodies' first source of energy is glucose. We get glucose from the foods that we eat. However, if we eat a low amount of carbs, then our bodies will have to get the energy it needs to continue functioning from somewhere else.

That somewhere else is going to be our fat stores. When we use fat for fuel instead of sugar, our bodies are in a state known as ketosis.

This is the state you want to be in when you're on the ketogenic diet. The main point of the ketogenic diet is to get your body to use fat as its main energy source instead of carbs.

The thing you have to remember is that, even if your body does adapt to using fat for fuel, this doesn't mean that things will always stay that way. For example, if your body has adapted to using fat for fuel, you still can't go back to eating a high amount of carbs.

If you do that, then you'll get kicked out of ketosis and go back to using sugar for fuel. By default, your body's first source of energy will be glucose.

If the glucose is present, then your body will use that for fuel first. This is why you must be committed to keeping your carb intake extremely low when it comes to a ketogenic diet; otherwise, the keto diet won't work for you.

However, keeping your carbs low isn't the only thing you have to be committed to when it comes to the ketogenic diet. You also have to eat a high amount of fat and a moderate amount of protein.

The reason why you have to eat a high amount of fat is that it will cause your body to produce more ketone bodies. The ketone bodies are going to be your body's new main source of fuel rather than glucose.

If you're not going to eat enough fat, then you're not going to produce enough ketone bodies. Not only that but if you're not eating enough fat, then that means you're either eating too many carbs or too much protein.

Eating too many carbs is bad for obvious reasons—you'll get kicked out of ketosis and have to use up that glucose before you can even think about getting back into that state.

However, eating too much protein is bad as well. Right now, you might not see the harm in eating a near equal amount of protein and fat in your diet.

For example, what would be so bad about eating 50% of your total calories from fat, 45% of your calories from protein, and 5% from carbs? Why does fat have to be higher and protein lower on a ketogenic diet?

Isn't protein supposed to be good for you? Yes, protein is good for you. It's very satiating, and it's responsible for repairing tissue, growing tissue, among other things.

However, you have to be careful that you don't over-consume it. The reason for this is that your body only needs so much protein on a daily basis.

With that being the case, what happens if you consume too much protein? What happens to the excess protein your body doesn't need?

It'll actually get converted into glucose via a process known as gluconeogenesis. This means that eating too much protein can actually end up kicking you out of ketosis.

While it may not sound like a good thing right now, if gluconeogenesis kicks in, it is for a good reason. It allows your body to keep functioning.

If you ever found yourself in a difficult situation like our ancestors did quite often, then your body would still have a way to get the energy it needs to continue sustaining your life, all thanks to processes such as gluconeogenesis.

So yes, there's a specific reason why you're eating the amount of fat, protein, and carbs that you are. It's all designed to help get your body into a state of ketosis so that you can use fat for fuel instead of carbs.

How Does the Dirty Keto Diet Differ From a Regular Ketogenic Diet?

So now that you know more of what a regular keto diet consists of, how does that differ from a dirty ketogenic diet? On a dirty ketogenic diet, you're still going to be consuming a high amount of fat, a moderate amount of protein, and a low amount of carbs.

Your primary goal is to get and stay in a state of ketosis, just like you would for the regular keto diet. A dirty ketogenic diet does not mean that you get to eat a higher amount of carbs, because that would defeat the purpose of the diet.

Instead, the main difference is the kind of foods that you'll be eating. On a regular or strict ketogenic diet, most of the foods you eat will be wholesome, organic foods.

For example, you would consume lots of vegetables that are high in fiber, various nuts and seeds, and organic butter. This is not to say that you can't consume these types of foods on a dirty keto diet because you certainly can if you want.

With a dirty keto diet, you may incorporate things such as artificial sweeteners, processed foods, and foods that are lower in fiber into your diet. Not everything you eat will be processed, but the difference is that processed foods are allowed on a dirty ketogenic diet, whereas the are not allowed on a strict keto diet.

Later on, I'll share with you the correct way to go about balancing the amount of clean and unclean foods you should eat on the dirty keto diet. There's a right and a wrong way to go about doing it, and you definitely don't want to mess it up.

Following a dirty ketogenic diet doesn't mean that you're allowed to eat whatever junk food you want, whenever you want, simply because it's low in carbs. There still needs to be a proper balance in place.

The main benefit of doing a dirty ketogenic diet is that it offers you more flexibility in your diet plan. This makes it much easier to do for a prolonged period of time.

You have to go into the dirty keto diet expecting to do it for years and years to come. If you don't, then your results will only last for as long as you're on the diet.

Most people have the wrong mentality when it comes to dieting. They try different diet plans in the hope of a quick fix. After they lose some weight, people often go back to their old way of eating, and then eventually they start to gain the weight back.

A lot of the time, this can be due to the fact that the diet plan was too restrictive or hard to keep up with. With the dirty keto diet, you're giving yourself some room to incorporate more of your favorite food choices, which makes it better for long-term sustainability.

What is Lazy Keto?

Another version of the keto diet is known as the lazy keto diet. Lazy keto doesn't deal with whether or not you'll eat strictly processed foods. Instead, it has more to do with tracking and measuring the foods that you eat.

On a ketogenic diet, it's critical that you know you're getting the right amount of fat, protein, and carbs. If you don't eat enough fat, then you might not be able to get into ketosis.

If you eat too much protein, then that extra protein could get converted to carbs via gluconeogenesis and kick you out of ketosis.

And finally, if you eat too many carbs, your body will continue to use sugar for energy instead of fat.

And if you have no idea of how much of each macro you're eating, then you're simply hoping for the best.

For this reason, I don't recommend the lazy keto diet if you are new to the ketogenic lifestyle.

You're still familiarizing yourself with what foods are keto approved and which ones aren't. You're still learning where carbs can be hidden in foods.

The last thing you want to do is take your best guess as to whether or not you're heading in the right direction. This is why you need to make sure you track every calorie and macro that you eat.

Don't worry, I'll show you exactly how to do that in a later chapter. And while I understand that this can be a pain in the neck, I promise that it's for your own good.

This will ensure that you're not wasting your time spinning your wheels. At the end of the day, you're following this diet plan because you want to get results.

Remember that you have to be diligent with the diet plan if you want to get those results. The good news is that you don't have to strictly track your calories and macros for the rest of your life.

As time goes on, you'll get better and better at knowing what foods you can and cannot eat. You'll know how many calories and macros certain foods contain.

This is a skill you'll acquire as time goes on. In the beginning though, you have to stay diligent with tracking your calories and macros. Unfortunately, there's no way of getting around this if you want to optimize your results and ensure that you're heading in the right direction.

Chapter 2: Caloric Intake and Macro Percentages on a Dirty Keto Diet

In this chapter, we're going to figure out exactly how many calories it is that you need to be eating every day. We're also going to figure out what percentage of each macro we'll be eating and then converting that into calories.

First though, it's important to understand how your body works in regards to weight loss.

How do you lose weight?

Every day, our bodies need energy. We get this energy from the foods that we eat.

Our bodies then take this energy and use it to fuel processes such as breathing and organ function. The exact amount of energy our bodies need to continue functioning is known as our resting metabolic rate.

For example, if someone burns off 1,800 calories a day, then his or her resting metabolic rate is 1,800 calories. What would happen if we were to eat more calories than our resting metabolic rate?

Our bodies would then store the excess energy as fat. And if we eat less than our bodies burn, then we'll use our stored fat for energy. For example:

Cindy's resting metabolic rate is 1,800 calories. Therefore:

- If Cindy eats more than 1,800 calories per day, she'll be in a caloric surplus and start to gain weight.
- If Cindy eats less than 1,800 calories per day, she'll start to lose weight.
- If Cindy eats right at 1,800 calories per day, then she'll neither gain nor lose weight.

The only way your body loses weight is by being in a caloric deficit. Even if you're on a ketogenic diet, you can still overeat on fat and not lose any weight.

This is why we want to make sure that we know how many calories it is that we need to eat. And even after you know that number, you still need to continue to track the amount of calories that you are eating.

Here's how you can figure out what your resting metabolic rate is:

Resting metabolic rate = Current bodyweight x13

For example, if Cindy currently weighs 138 pounds, she'll take 138 and multiply it by 13 to get 1,800 calories per day. If Cindy wants to lose weight, she needs to eat less than 1,800 calories per day.

The question becomes how large of a caloric deficit should you aim to create? If you create too large of a deficit, then it'll make the diet plan harder to sustain for the long-term.

Sure you'll get results fast, but you'll end up crashing and burning. On the other hand, you don't want to create too small of a deficit.

It'll be easy to maintain, but you won't be losing weight at any considerable pace. Therefore, the best way to go about things is to go in the middle of these two extremes.

You want to aim for around 1 pound of fat loss per week. That might not seem like a lot, but remember we're talking about pure fat loss here.

This will add up to make a much bigger difference than you think. Losing even 5 pounds of fat can have a profound impact on how you look, but imagine losing 52 pounds of fat in one year!

That would make a big difference. I want to mention that you're more than likely going to lose more than one pound per week when you first get started on the ketogenic diet.

This is mostly going to be water weight. The reason people lose a lot of water weight when they first get started is that for every gram of glycogen you eat, the body will also store 3-4 grams of water.

Now that you won't be consuming any more carbs, your body will also be getting rid of that extra stored water. And since water isn't massless, the number on the scale will go down.

Remember though, it's not water loss that we're after here. The main thing we care about is fat loss. So after you've been on the keto diet for a few weeks, the main goal is going to be losing 1 pound of fat per week.

And since there are 3,500 calories in one pound of fat (1), this means you need to create a cumulative weekly caloric deficit of 3,500 calories in order to burn one pound of fat per week.

If you take 3,500 and divide it by 7 days in the week, this comes out to a total of 500 calories per day. Therefore to lose one pound of fat per week, you need to create an average daily deficit of 500 calories. Here's how to factor that in with your resting metabolic rate, using Cindy as an example:

Resting metabolic rate = 1,800 calories

1,800-500 = 1,300

Therefore Cindy needs to eat 1,300 calories per day in order to burn one pound of fat per week.

Calories aren't the only thing we need to be concerned with. We also have to track the amount of fat, carbs, and protein that we consume as well. These are the macronutrient percentages that we're going to be consuming on this dirty ketogenic diet:

Fat: 75% of our total daily calories
Protein: 20% of our total daily calories
Carbs: 5% of our total daily calories

Here's how to factor these macro percentages into your daily caloric intake:

1,300x.75 = 975 calories from fat
1,300x.2 = 260 calories from protein
1,300x.05 = 65 calories from carbs

You can then determine the gram equivalent by doing the following, since there are 9 calories per gram of fat and 4 calories per gram of protein and carbohydrate:

975/9 = 108.33 grams of fat per day
260/4 = 65 grams of protein per day
65/4 = 16.25 grams of carbs per day

How to Track Your Calorie and Macro Percentages

The next thing you need to do once you've calculated your calories and macro percentages is to actually track them. The easiest way to go about doing this is to use an app on your smartphone.

Simply type in "macro calculator" or "calorie calculator" and download one that you like. Most of them have similar features so it's hard to go wrong.

Once you have an app, the next thing you want to do is log all of the calories that you eat in the app. Most of the apps have barcode scanners, allowing you to easily scan and log whatever it is that you eat automatically.

You can also type in the food that you're eating, and log the nutritional information that way as well. The one thing you will need to know is the portion size of the foods that you're eating.

This is where something such as a food scale will come in handy. You will be able to know exactly how much of a certain food you're eating so you can determine the proper amount of calories and macros contained in it.

Even though modern technology will make tracking your calories and macros much easier, it's still a skill that you'll get better with as time goes on. Initially, you must be patient with yourself.

Now there will also be some times where you're not going to know exactly how many calories a certain food contains. For example, you might be at a party where one of your friends made a special recipe, and you have no idea what any of the nutritional information is.

In cases such as these, you're simply going to take your best guess as to how many calories are contained in that food. Obviously, since you're on a keto diet, you first and foremost need to make sure that it doesn't contain carbs.

After that, you're going to have to eyeball and guess how many calories the dish contains. This isn't easy by any means, especially considering the fact that you won't know how much protein or fat the dish contains either.

All you can do is take your best guess and move on. Do whatever you can to try and figure out the caloric and macro content of the dish.

Ultimately though, if you can't find that out, then you'll have to take your best guess. This can get you into trouble, as most people go about the eyeball test the wrong way.

They tend to underestimate the number of calories they eat. You don't want to do this because that can cause you to overeat.

For example, if your friend's dish contained 500 calories per serving and you estimated that it contained 300 calories, then you'll end up eating an extra 200 calories that you shouldn't have.

That's why it's much better to overestimate how many calories are contained in the foods you're unsure of. In this case, it'd be much better to estimate that the dish contained 700 calories even though in reality it only contained 500.

Sure you're still overshooting, but at least now you'll eat 200 fewer calories than you were supposed to at the end of the day. This will still allow you to be in a caloric deficit, meaning you won't lose any progress as you work towards your weight loss goals.

For the most part though, most of the things you eat will be easy to track and measure.

As time goes on, you'll easily be able to track the meals that you regularly eat because you'll already know the nutritional information.

It's just a matter of being patient with yourself as you get used to tracking your calories and macros. It can be a tedious thing to do at first, but it's well worth it to know that you're on the right track!

Chapter 3: Why Most Fail with Keto and What You Can Do to Be Different

It shouldn't come as a surprise that most people aren't successful when it comes to dieting. This holds true for the ketogenic diet.

Most people who start a ketogenic diet ultimately won't be successful with it for the long-term. And if we're being honest, long-term results are the only thing that matter.

If you lose 20 pounds on the ketogenic diet, and then you gain it all back 2 months later, what good did it do you? In this chapter, you're going to learn why it is that most people fail when it comes to dieting, and what you can do to ensure that you'll be different.

The Typical Dieting Mindset

Most people fail before a diet plan even begins. This can be for one of two main reasons—either the diet plan is setting people up for failure, or the person going on the diet has the wrong mentality.

Many of the mainstream diets are terrible, and they set people up to fail right from the start. An example of this would be something like a crash diet where the dieter would only be eating 500 calories per day.

This isn't going to end well for the person on the diet and rebound weight gain is going to occur. The other problem that often causes failure is the mindset of the individual.

Many people start a diet with the hope of a quick fix. They want to lose weight as fast as possible, but they don't have much of a plan for what they'll do once they lose the weight. Impatience is the real issue here.

You didn't gain all of the excess weight overnight, and you can't expect to lose it all overnight either. That's why it's better to think of things as a lifestyle change instead of a diet.

When someone says that he or she is going on a diet, this means that eventually that person will go off that diet. Whenever that happens, he or she will start to gain the weight back.

The phrase "going on a diet" implies the short-term. It means doing something miserable for as long as you can handle it.

When you finally can't take it anymore, you quit and go back to your old way of eating. Instead of doing this, think of things in terms of a lifestyle change.

This phrase implies permanent change for the rest of your life. This has a much more powerful impact on your subconscious mind.

Now making something a lifestyle change doesn't mean eating 500 calories a day and calling that a lifestyle change instead of a diet. It means doing things in a way that makes whatever nutrition plan you're doing sustainable for the long haul.

And in the case of the dirty ketogenic diet, that's exactly what we're doing. On the strict ketogenic diet for example, if you drank a diet soda, you'd technically be breaking the rules of the diet.

This could make you feel like a failure and make you want to quit the plan. However, this would still be allowed on the dirty keto diet, making it much easier to follow.

If drinking a diet soda every now and again helps you keep your sanity and allows you to keep on marching forward, then by all means do it. That's just one example of course, but implementing a proper lifestyle change comes down to striking a balance between structure and flexibility.

If a nutrition plan is too rigid, then you won't be able to keep up with it for years and years to come. On the other hand, if you have too much flexibility, then you might not end up with enough guidelines that'll allow you to get results.

Your diet plan could look similar to your old way of eating simply because there are no rules for your new nutrition plan. Thankfully, the dirty ketogenic diet will allow you to have a nice balance between structure and flexibility.

You have rules for certain things that you're not going to be able to eat (such as carbohydrates). Yet, these rules aren't so strict that it feels like you're in prison.

Throughout the rest of this book, I'm still going to be using the word diet in the normal sense that you're used to. From now on though, when you hear the word diet, I don't want you to think about it in the short-term 'get quick results' way that most people do.

I want you to view it more as a long-term permanent change because that's the only way that you'll truly be successful.

How to Stop Emotional Eating

Another thing that holds a lot of people back when on the ketogenic diet is the 'emotional eating' habit, which is when you eat to distract yourself from a certain feeling or emotion, as opposed to eating because you are truly hungry.

This can be especially dangerous on the ketogenic diet because you may binge eat on something that contains a lot of carbs, which means you'll get kicked out of ketosis. And most of the time "comfort foods" such as potato chips and ice cream are some of the first things people reach for when they eat out of emotion.

These foods are high in fat and sugar, which take energy from our nervous system and transfer it to the digestive system. This is why eating these kinds of foods can literally make us feel temporarily numb to whatever emotion it is that we're feeling.

And once someone gets kicked out of ketosis, it can be a slippery slope for a lot of people from that point forward. Once you've eaten a lot of carbs, it's easy to say to yourself, "Well I already got kicked out of ketosis, I might as well eat whatever it is that I want!"

The thing about this is that one meal can turn into one day, which turns into 2 days, which turns into a week or longer without ever getting back on track. That's why it's so important to recognize when you're eating out of emotion instead of hunger.

The reality is that we eat food to nourish our bodies and to get energy. We don't need to eat to cope with a certain emotion that we're feeling.

There are other ways to cope that don't involve eating too many calories. So what should you do if you know you eat out of emotion sometimes?

The first thing and most important thing that you can do is to be aware. You want to first and foremost notice what emotion it is that you're feeling whenever you binge eat some ice cream, for example.

When you catch yourself eating something like ice cream, ask yourself "What emotion am I trying to run away from right now?" It could be sadness, anger, fear, or something else.

Most of us think that it's not okay to experience saddening emotions. The truth is that it is perfectly fine and normal to feel these things.

In fact, we wouldn't know what happiness truly felt like if we weren't able to compare it to sadness. While it is okay to feel these things at times, it's not okay to bury the emotion and try to forget about it.

It will resurface, and it needs to be addressed. You could have experienced something as a child, and when something triggers you, it brings back that emotion you felt as a kid.

For example, a woman might fear that a man will never truly love her. Maybe she feels this way because her father was never around in her life growing up as a child.

These feelings might carry over into her adult life. When she starts dating, someone might text her and cancel the date on her and not give much of a reason why.

She'll feel like her date canceled because no man will ever love her. The reality is that her date could've gotten busy at work or something else came up, and he had to cancel.

However, that doesn't matter because that's not the story the woman is telling herself. Instead, she might go home and binge eat to help cope with her feelings of sadness.

Soon afterwards though, she'll feel even worse than before because she knows that she ate a lot of something she shouldn't have, and now she feels unloved, guilty, and bloated.

This can cause more feelings of sadness and hopelessness, which can lead to more emotional eating. This is why the cycle can be so vicious and hard to break through.

So in this case, what should this woman do to break out of her habit of emotional eating? She should first recognize that she wants to binge eat.

Then she needs to ask herself, why am I feeling the way that I am right now? She would then come to realize that it's because her date canceled on her.

This is a good start, but it's not deep enough. She needs to ask herself why it is that she's so upset about the situation.

Yes, it's understandable to be upset, but why is she going into a complete tailspin over this? She needs to think of moments from her past and see if there's any reason why she might be feeling this way.

At that point, she might realize that she never really felt loved by her father. This could be the reason why she's feeling insecure when someone cancels a date.

Figuring this out is very powerful. She can now break the cycle because of this awareness. It wouldn't be enough to simply be aware though.

You must find a way to be able to handle the emotion instead of trying to bury it away. In this case, communication would be the key.

She would need to make sure that she gets a good explanation for why her date canceled and see if they can reschedule. She can't assume that her date canceled because no one will ever love her.

She has to challenge those original assumptions and see if there's any truth to them. In this case, just because her father wasn't around doesn't mean that there won't be a good guy for her to date.

Even if someone would completely stand her up, that wouldn't mean it was her fault. The guy could simply be a jerk who has his own problems he's dealing with.

This is what she would need to understand and recognize so that she can feel confident in who she is as a person. Another example might be someone who eats because he's bored.

In this case, he would need to figure out when and where it is that he eats out of boredom. He may realize that he eats when he watches television at home.

If nothing good is on at the moment, he might eat as a way to make up for the boring shows. If this is the case, then he needs to find something different to do other than watching TV.

Maybe he could start a game night with his friends, read a book, or learn a new skill. Essentially, he would need to do something else that would help distract him and help him keep his mind off of food.

Even if he's aware of the problem, that might not be enough. As soon as he starts to get bored again, he may reach for the potato chips without even realizing it. The best thing he can do is stay as busy as possible or else the cycle will keep repeating itself.

What Can You Do to Become More Aware?

This information might sound great, but how can you become more aware if most of the time you don't catch yourself emotionally eating? Thankfully, there are a couple of different things that you can do.

The first one is to start asking yourself *why* you ate after every meal you eat. For example, if you normally eat dinner at 7:00, then you'll know you ate because that's when you usually eat.

However, if you got a snack at the vending machine, then ask yourself why you ate that candy bar. Were you actually hungry? Or are you trying to distract yourself from your work?

You have to ask yourself why after every meal you eat for the sake of consistency. This will help you make it into a habit, making it more likely that you'll be able to catch yourself when you're eating out of emotion.

The next thing that you can do is set an alarm for the end of the day. When the alarm goes off, think about what all you ate for the day, and why it was that you ate those things.

Did the soap opera really make the ice cream taste that much better, or are you stressed out at work? Did you get fast food because you truly wanted it, or because you're worn out and tired after a long day?

Finally, the most effective thing you can do is keep a food log. Basically, you'll log everything that you eat and also write what emotion you were feeling when you ate that food.

For example, if you ate some ice cream, you would log that you ate ice cream at 9:00 and that you were feeling sad. This is how you'll be able to become more aware of whether or not you're emotionally eating.

How to Stop Binge Eating

The next thing that trips a lot of people up on the ketogenic diet is binge eating. The reason why this happens is because people may have the wrong mentality.

For example, the person might be at a work event where lots of delicious non-ketogenic foods are being served. If the person eats something that isn't ketogenic, then he might feel that he can eat whatever he wants now because he already ruined his diet plan.

This is especially true on the ketogenic diet. Once someone eats more carbs than he should have, then the person feels that he might as well eat whatever he wants since he's already been kicked out of ketosis.

The thing is though, once you get kicked out of ketosis, you might not continue following the diet because of how long it'll take you to get back into ketosis. The next day you might wake up and think, "Well I'm already out of ketosis so I might as well eat how I please today."

If you do that for another day, it only makes it that much harder to get back on track with the ketogenic diet. And before you know it, it could be weeks or months since you've last eaten keto.

Binge eating is a problem with any diet plan; however, it's especially something that you'll want to be aware of when you're on the ketogenic diet. Being in ketosis is the main point of the ketogenic diet.

While it makes sense that people would eat however they please when they are out of ketosis, it's important to resist the temptation. Like I mentioned earlier, this could create a vicious cycle where long amounts of time go by before you get back on track. Think of it like working out in the gym.

Let's say you have a schedule to workout 5 days a week after you get off work. On Wednesday, you're really tired, and you decide to go home instead of going to the gym.

Then when Thursday rolls around, do you think it's going to be easier or harder to go to the gym after work? It's going to be a little bit harder because you skipped yesterday.

And if you skip your workout on Thursday, then it's going to be that much easier to skip on Friday. Then the next thing you know it'll be weeks before you go back.

Now consider the opposite scenario. If you workout on Monday, you will create momentum that will make it slightly easier for you to go on Tuesday. Then if you workout on Tuesday, that will make it a little bit easier to go on Wednesday.

The same is true for the ketogenic diet. Every day that you do the ketogenic diet will make it that much easier for you to continue doing it.

Each day you don't follow the ketogenic diet will make it that much harder to get back into it. Thinking of this ahead of time will help you out.

For example, let's say you've been following the dirty ketogenic diet for 3 weeks without any problems. Then you're at an office party and you're surrounded by a bunch of delicious carbs.

Before you decide to eat anything you know you shouldn't, you can think about how you'll be breaking your streak of 3 weeks. You can then think about how hard it'll be to get back in the groove of eating a ketogenic diet and ask yourself if that moment of glory will truly be worth it.

In most cases, it won't be. It'll likely bring up feelings of guilt and potentially lead to you spiraling out of control and eating whatever you want. Not only that, but these cravings of certain carbs that you may have will come and go.

As time goes on, you won't crave these foods like you used to. However, let's say you did eat something you feel you shouldn't have.

What should you do in these cases? For example, let's say you ate a brownie and ice cream at the party.

First and foremost, you must stop the bleeding. Think about what you do when you get a cut. Do you say to yourself, "I'm bleeding! I guess I might as well keep on bleeding until I've bled a good amount."

No, of course you don't say that. Instead, when you start bleeding, you apply pressure and a bandage in order to stop the bleeding.

You don't want things to get any worse than they already are. Sadly, when it comes to binge eating, most people have the kind of attitude as if they should keep bleeding!

If you ate something high in carbs, then you might as well splurge and eat to your heart's content. Of course, that is the wrong attitude to have.

Instead, you're much better off stopping the bleeding. If you ate a brownie and ice cream, then leave it at that.

Don't use getting kicked out of ketosis as an excuse to eat whatever you want for the rest of the day. Remember that the more carbs you eat, the longer it's going to take to burn off those carbs, thus making it that much longer for you to get back into ketosis.

Even if you ate something that kicked you out of ketosis, you can stop the bleeding and get back in it that much sooner if you don't binge eat everything in sight. Continuing to eat will only make the feelings of guilt and regret that much harder to overcome.

This leads me to my next point, which is that you have to understand that mistakes will happen. You're human, and you're not perfect. Going into this dirty ketogenic diet, the idea is to limit your carbohydrate intake to 5% of your total calories.

Doing that every single day for the rest of your life would mean that you did things perfectly. However, there are very few people who would be able to diligently follow a diet plan 100% of the time.

There might be moments where you eat too many carbs. That's okay as long as you pick yourself back up and keep on moving forward.

The only thing that can stop you is you. If you make a mistake and eat too many carbs, you have one of two choices.

You can admit to yourself that you're human and things like this will happen at times, or you can quit and go back to your old habits of eating.

If you choose the latter, then you're guaranteed to not get any more results. Embracing the fact that things won't always go smoothly will make it easier to move on from mistakes whenever they do happen.

Most people don't do that though. They tell themselves that things have to go perfectly. This creates an image in your mind that you'll never slip up and eat something that you're not supposed to.

When you do eat something you're not supposed to, then you're not acting in a way that's consistent with what you told yourself. This is what leads to feelings of guilt, frustration, and ultimately leads to you quitting.

Then you'll go back to your old eating habits because it's easy to stay perfect when you're eating whatever it is that you please. Instead, if you tell yourself that you will slip up at times, then you'll still be consistent with your beliefs when something does go wrong. This'll make it much easier to move past it.

How to Use Implementation Intention to Increase Your Chances of Success

What typically happens when people start a new diet or exercise plan? People say that they're going to do something, but then they struggle to actually do it.

Saying that you're going to do something and thinking about doing it usually isn't enough for people to be able to consistently follow through. This is where a technique known as implementation intention comes in handy.

Implementation intention is where you write down the conditions of completing a certain task. One study compared three different groups. The first group was told to follow an exercise routine for the next two weeks. The second group was told the same thing, and they were also shown videos about the benefits of exercise.

The final group was also told to exercise and watch the videos; in addition, the final group was told to write down by their own hand that they would exercise, including the specific time and place for when and where they would exercise.

The results didn't find much of a difference in exercise adherence between the first and second group. However, the third group was more than twice as likely to stick to the exercise plan in comparison to the other two groups (2).

Those are some pretty crazy results considering the fact that all you have to do is write a simple sentence. What makes writing that one sentence so powerful?

It comes down to something known as decision fatigue. We only have so much willpower to make decisions with. As the day goes on, our willpower starts to drain.

Once it's drained, your ability to start the things you know you should do (such as exercise or eating healthier) goes way down. In fact, it's even been said that the decision to workout takes more willpower than it does to actually do the workout itself.

This is why you'll see successful people wear the same thing every day. It allows them to not have to waste their precious deciding power on a trivial decision such as what to wear for the day.

Instead, they can save their willpower for much more important decisions later on in the day. With implementation intention, you're essentially doing the same thing as a successful businessman who wears the same thing every day.

You're already deciding ahead of time what it is that you're going to do when you're fresh. So how can you use implementation intention to increase your chances of success with the dirty ketogenic diet?

You can use it to plan out your meals ahead of time. For example, you could write down and say something along the lines of, "I eat three ketogenic meals at 8:00 a.m., 1:00 p.m., and 6:00 p.m. I eat two of my meals at home and one meal while I'm at work."

This will now give you specific times and places for which you'll eat at. Now you won't have to think about it every day because it's already been decided ahead of time for you.

The cool thing is that you can even take this one step farther by meal prepping. Don't worry, I cover how to go about doing this more in the chapter dedicated to meal prepping, but it really can be the difference between success and failure.

And it all comes back down to decision fatigue. Imagine this scenario, which will be happening more often than not.

You come home from work and want to eat a ketogenic meal. Then you realize that you don't have the groceries you need in order to make that meal.

In order to make this meal, you'd have to go to the store, buy the groceries, cook the meal, eat it, and clean up any dirty dishes afterwards. That's going to sound very overwhelming considering the fact that you just got home from work.

Instead, it'd be much easier to go and grab some fast food. All you have to do is drive through and pick up the food, eat it once you get home, and you're good to go.

There's nothing to clean up afterwards. In this situation, it could take more willpower to decide to make a healthy ketogenic meal than it could to actually make the meal. And like I mentioned, this is something you're going to be dealing with on most days.

It can make it hard to be successful for the long haul if you're not properly planning ahead. With meal prepping ahead of time, you can save yourself from constantly having to think about what you're going to eat, and then going through all of the effort to make the meal.

Consider the fact that if you eat three meals a day, then that means you're going to decide 3 times a day what it is you're going to eat if you take it meal-by-meal. This means you're making 21 independent decisions on what to eat throughout the week.

If you meal prep, you can cut that down considerably. You can decide on one day what all of your 21 meals will be for the week.

Now you're batching that to one day or two days, depending on how you want to meal prep. For example, imagine that on Sunday you plan ahead and prepare all of your meals for the week.

You would plan out all of the meals that you're going to eat. Then you would go to the grocery store and buy those groceries.

You would come home and batch cook for all of the meals. Now when Wednesday night rolls around and you're tired, you don't have to think.

The decision has already been made for you ahead of time when you weren't fatigued. All you have to do is take out the meal that you're going to eat, heat it up in the microwave, and you'll be good to go.

This seriously is my favorite tip to help increase your chances of success on the ketogenic diet. As far as implementation intention is concerned, you could write down the following sentence, "I meal prep all of my meals for the upcoming week on Sunday's starting at 2:00 p.m."

And don't worry, you can write down more than one sentence using the implementation intention technique. In this case, you'd be writing down how many meals you're going to eat per day, and what time you're going to eat them at.

You'd also be writing down when you're going to be preparing those meals to drastically increase your chances of success. Not only that, but if you want to add in exercise, then you could use implementation intention for that as well.

You could write down something along the lines of, "I do a 30-minute cardio workout on Monday, Wednesday, and Friday at 5:00 p.m." Essentially, any new habit that you're trying to form can benefit from using this technique of implementation intention..

And you're not limited to using it solely for your health and fitness goals. Use it for other areas of your life such as relationship and financial goals.

For example, you could say something like, "I review my financial statement once per week every Sunday at 7:00 p.m." Or for your relationship, you could say, "I take my spouse out on a date every Saturday starting at 6:00 p.m."

Finally, I want to give you a few more tips to ensure that you maximize the potential of implementation intention. Firstly, I recommend that you write it down using pen and paper.

Don't just think about it in your head or even type it. When you physically write something down it, makes it far more real than just another idea in your head that you'll eventually get around to.

You're much more engaged in the process when you write down what it is that you intend to do. The next thing you'll notice is that we're writing these sentences down in the present tense.

This helps to create a greater sense of urgency; if you say "I *will* do. . . " then it makes it easier to keep delaying the thing you know you should do. Finally, don't just write it down once and forget about it.

This technique becomes more powerful the more you write down your processes. For optimal results, write down all of the processes you're going to do morning and night.

This way it'll be the first thing on your mind and the last thing on your mind before you go to bed at night. Also, be sure to keep a copy of your implementation intention sentences at a place where you'll regularly see them.

For example, this could mean keeping a copy of them by your desk at work. This way they'll always be on the front of your mind and thus increase the chances of you following through.

The Importance of Self-Image

The next thing I want to talk about is self-image and its importance in regards to your success on the dirty ketogenic diet. Self-image is basically the way you view and think about yourself in regards to different things.

A lot of these beliefs are deep in our subconscious mind, and it affects our daily decisions. Let's use the example of money. Many of us grow up with the belief that money is hard to come by.

We're told that money doesn't grow on trees, and we act as if money is a scarce resource. If that's what we believe about money, then how hard do you think money will be to come by?

The decisions we make and how we spend it will be affected by our viewpoints on money. Another example might be someone who is shy. Maybe when growing up, this person was told by his parents and schoolteachers that he was a shy child.

Now that this person is an adult, he doesn't go out much or meet new people because he labels himself as in introvert. As long as he holds that image of being an introvert, he won't go out and meet new people for example.

He must change the way he views himself in order break out of his shyness. Finally consider two different people, each with a scar on his face.

The first person could be a war hero who sees his wound as a battle scar and is proud of the scar because it represents what he's been through. The other person might be a salesman who got into a car accident, and now his confidence is ruined because this scar is not in congruence with how he views himself.

He views himself as a handsome, well put together man. He thinks the scar makes him look less handsome; therefore, his confidence is shaken. The way he views his scar will now affect him in how he makes sales.

The subconscious mind is very powerful. It doesn't understand the difference between something that's actually happening versus something that's being vividly imagined or perceived.

Think about what we do when we worry about something. We think about something negative happening in the future and our minds think that thing is really happening or about to happen.

And if we worry enough about something, it ends up actually happening most of the time.

Our brain is like a supercomputer. It'll act on the information that we give it. Therefore, we can also feed our mind positive thoughts and outcomes, and our mind will perceive it as being real just like it does when we worry.

If we're going to think about the future, we might as well think about it in a more positive way. Using the example from earlier, the "shy person" could imagine himself having a fun and meaningful conversation with someone he just met.

However, chances are good that he probably doesn't think of having conversations with strangers in this way. He'll probably imagine himself being awkward, or not knowing what to say next; therefore, that may very be what ends up happening.

So how does all of this relate to fitness? Well, if your self-image is that of being overweight, then it doesn't matter what you do to lose weight.

Ultimately, you'll find a way to sabotage yourself and gain all of the weight back. It might seem random, but eventually you'll go back to the old self-image you have of yourself as being an overweight person.

Therefore, if the self-image doesn't change, then neither will your results. Regardless of how good this dirty keto diet plan is, you must change your self-image to that of the person you want to be.

You might not think that developing your self –image is important, and that we should focus purely on the diet itself instead. That would be a mistake because dieting isn't a purely mechanical process.

It's not as simple as me telling you what to do and then you going out and doing it. Ultimately, if you don't have the right mindset and self-image, then you won't be successful regardless of what your nutrition plan is. Now let's get into how you can actually go about changing your self-image.

How to Change Your Self-Image

In order to be able to change your self-image, you must first be able to understand what forms it in the first place. Your self-image is shaped by your past experiences.

Using our previous example of the shy person, maybe when he was a kid his parents introduced him as being shy. Unfortunately, his parents likely had no idea that they were ingraining this belief into their child.

Or maybe this person had a bad experience and was humiliated by an adult when he tried to speak up about something. That experience taught him that it's better to keep quiet rather than to speak up and be made a fool of.

Now because of these experiences, he labels himself as a shy person. That's just who he is. However, is that really true?

Will his past shyness mean that he'll always be shy for the rest of his life and that he'll never be able to become more social? Of course not!

That's why the first step that you must take when it comes to changing your self-image is to question the belief in the first place. As a matter of fact, when circuses are training elephants, they'll tether one of the elephant's feet to a pole.

When they first do this, the elephant is young and unable to break free from the rope. What's interesting is that, as time goes on, they'll use the same measly rope to tether a giant, fully grown elephant.

The elephant won't even try to break free. It's obvious to anyone who sees the elephant that it could easily break free from the rope if it simply tried to do so. We must not be like an elephant in the circus; instead, we must question the validity of our beliefs.

For example, if you've struggled to maintain a healthy body weight for most of your life, does that really mean you're destined to stay that way for the remainder of your life? Of course it doesn't.

I'm sure you might consciously know that right now as you read this; however, that's not what matters most. What matters most are the beliefs that are deeply held in your subconscious mind.

Until we can root out those myths that were planted in your subconscious mind, nothing will change. Most people know that they need to diet and exercise in order to lose weight, and yet most people aren't successful when it comes to dieting.

And the reason for that is because most people have a poor self-image. They don't believe that they're worthy of getting in shape.

And the first thing you need to do to make yourself feel worthy is to *act* worthily. Think about how you would act if you were already at your goal bodyweight.

What would your posture look like? What thoughts would you think? Would you give yourself positive or negative self-talk?

You must start to act and think as if you're already at your goal bodyweight. Right now you might be thinking, "Thomas, this sounds great and all, but it's hard for me to think of myself in a positive way when I know it's not true. It makes me feel like I'm a fraud."

In response to that, I would say it's okay if you feel that way. What you need to do is attach something you already believe about yourself to your new thoughts.

For example, let's say you're really good at planning and organizing. This skill would greatly help you out because you'll be able to meal prep on this diet.

You could then tell yourself, "I'm fit and healthy because of my ability to plan out my meals ahead of time." This is much more powerful than simply saying, "I'm fit and healthy." and having your subconscious mind balk at the idea of that.

Another example could be that you're a morning person. You might be the type of person who wakes up early seven days a week just because you like to.

If that's the case then great, you can wake up early and prepare a healthy meal or exercise with the time you have instead of waking up and feeling rushed. You could tell yourself something like, "I'm at a healthy body weight because I'm a morning person."

You might have to dig deeper than others to find something, but don't skip on this exercise. It doesn't have to be some grand thing. You could say that you're diligent, always on time, meticulous when it comes to small details, or some other positive habit, and relate that back to your new self-image. This will make the exercise much more powerful and believable to your subconscious mind.

The second thing you must do to rewire your subconscious mind is to use visualization. Remember what I said earlier—your subconscious mind doesn't know the difference between something that's actually happening versus something that's being vividly imagined.

Therefore, by using visualization you can make your subconscious mind think that this is really the way things are. And you don't have to practice this for very long.

Even just a few minutes a day will give you great benefits. For example, you could visualize yourself being at your goal bodyweight for two minutes when you wake up and another two minutes before you go to bed.

You could even do five minutes in the morning and five minutes in the evening if you want. The main point is to be consistent with it.

When you do your visualization, get really vivid with it. Make your visualizations really detailed. Involve all of your senses.

This will make the exercise much more effective. For example, what foods are you eating? What do they smell like? What do they taste like? What are your energy levels like throughout the day? What do you think you'll feel like when you're at your goal bodyweight?

Imagine yourself talking to your friends and family and them giving you compliments. Picture exactly what you'll look like and what clothes you'll wear.

You want to get as detailed with this as you possibly can. Now, it's important to mention that you must be patient with this. When you first start, your mind will tend to wander a lot.

Don't beat yourself up when you notice this happening. Instead, gently guide your mind back to the main focus, which is the visualization.

As time goes on, you'll get better and better at it, so keep at it. Thirdly, you need to shift the focus. Through these exercises, you're starting to develop a new identity of who you are.

You're starting to develop a better version of yourself. However, this doesn't mean that there won't be bumps along the way. You'll still make mistakes.

The important thing is to be careful not to let the mistakes trip you up when they do happen. When you make a mistake or do something that's incongruent with your new self, your mind won't hesitate to let you know about it.

Thoughts such as, "I knew I wasn't cut out for this", or "I knew this wouldn't last for long" are undoubtedly going to pop into your mind. Don't worry if this happens to you because it's completely normal.

Your mind is still being resistant to the idea of this new version of yourself. You must catch yourself when you notice that you're thinking these negative thoughts.

Awareness is the key here. Most people aren't even aware of what they're thinking and how it affects them. You must be different.

You must start becoming more aware of your thoughts. You'll start to notice patterns of things that upset you and start a downward spiral.

What you can do to stop a negative thought pattern? is Anchor an image of something in your head that symbolizes you needing to halt. For example, when you catch yourself thinking negative thoughts, think of something such as a big red stop sign.

This will signal you to stop thinking those thoughts. Over time, this will get more ingrained in you, and you'll get better and better at it as time goes on.

Once the negative thoughts have stopped, the next thing that you need to do is replace those negative thoughts with some positive ones. For example, you can think of some things that you've done right during the week.

Maybe on Sunday you did a good job of planning and preparing your meals for the week. When Monday comes around, you can think about how you followed through and ate everything according to the plan.

Finally, the last thing you can do to help improve your self-image is to write down your visualizations. When you're visualizing how you want to look and feel after successfully going on this dirty keto diet, write every detail of the visualization.

Writing it down will help to make things even more real for your subconscious mind. Once you're done writing it down, be sure to look at it regularly.

Really feel everything that you wrote down as you read over it. Look for similarities that are in the visualization and compare them to how you're actually living your life.

Also look for incongruencies between what you wrote down and how you're living. Use these differences to help you improve.

Improving your self-image may seem tedious and unnecessary. However, the rest of the information in this book about the dirty ketogenic diet is meaningless if you don't feel that you're worthy of being fit and achieving success.

Therefore, don't gloss over the exercises in this chapter; take them to heart and really practice them. Following through with these exercises could really make a difference in whether or not you find success on this diet.

Are you enjoying this book so far? If so, please consider leaving a review. Even just a few words would help others decide if the book is right for them. Many thanks in advance!

Chapter 4: How to Overcome the Keto Flu

One thing that people commonly experience on the ketogenic diet is something known as the keto flu. Common symptoms of the keto flu include things such as fatigue, weakness, body aches, headaches, food cravings, and brain fog, among others.

The keto flu will usually occur within the first few days of you starting the diet, and it can last for days or even weeks in some cases. You might think that the keto flu is a necessary evil that you have to put up with, but as it turns out, that may not be the case. . .

What Causes the Keto Flu?

It's important to understand what exactly causes the keto flu to begin with. You have to remember that we're trying to make our bodies become 'fat adapted,' meaning our bodies use fat for fuel instead of carbs.

With the ketogenic diet, we want our bodies to get the energy it needs from ketone bodies, not from glucose. In order to achieve that, you must lower your carbohydrate intake and increase your fat intake.

As your body starts to lose glucose, it's also going to lose a lot of water. For every gram of carbohydrate that is stored in your body, your body will also store 2-3 grams of water along with it.

This means that when you start shedding those stored carbs, you're also going to be shedding even more water along with it. And since you're losing water, this means that you're going to be losing a lot of key electrolytes such as sodium, magnesium, and potassium.

Having a lowered amount of electrolytes in the body is what causes the keto flu to occur. Therefore, the keto flu isn't something you just have to put up with as your body starts to become fat adapted.

Instead, you can actually prevent it from occurring in the first place with the proper game plan. You'll now know ahead of time that your body is going to start losing a lot of these key electrolytes, so you can beat the keto flu to the punch by taking measures to replace the electrolytes that you're going to lose.

Even if you're not able to completely prevent these keto flu symptoms from happening, you'll know what to do if they start to occur. Obviously, I recommend that you start eating the necessary foods or taking a supplement right out of the gate when you start the ketogenic diet.

This will give you the best chance at preventing the keto flu from happening in the first place. However, if some symptoms do start to come up, then the following will help you know exactly which electrolyte could be the problem.

Sodium

This one might be hard for people to wrap their heads around because sodium generally has a bad reputation. Consuming too much sodium can be a bad thing.

Excess sodium can lead to an increase in blood pressure because you'll be holding onto excessive amounts of water. And increased blood pressure can lead to a heart attack or stroke.

On the typical American diet, people are consuming an excessive amount of sodium due to poor food choices. Not only that, but these poor food choices also contain a lot of carbs, which will make it easier for the body to retain sodium.

While too much sodium can be harmful, it also has some important functions in the body. You wouldn't want to completely get rid of it—that would be very bad!

For example, sodium helps regulate blood pressure levels. If you've ever stood up and felt light-headed, it could be because you have a low amount of sodium in your body.

Sodium is also necessary for nerve and muscle function as well as helping the body regulate the amount of water found in and around the cells. So what should you be on the lookout for to see if your body is losing too much sodium once you cut carbs?

Common symptoms of low sodium include lightheadedness upon standing up, nausea, dizziness, or muscle cramps.

So what can you do to increase your sodium intake? The first thing you might be thinking of right now is table salt, which would certainly be an easy way to increase your sodium intake.

However, I want to caution you as to what kind of salt you decide to use. Yes, this is a dirty ketogenic diet, meaning you can consume things like regular table salt and be just fine.

Even with that being the case, I want to make a plea for you to consider using something such as pink Himalayan salt or Celtic sea salt. Regular table salt is purified using a manufacturing process that heats the salt at 1,200 degrees Fahrenheit.

This process leaves you with roughly 97.5% sodium chloride and 2.5% of additives. These additives include various things such as caking agents to help prevent the salt from sticking together.

It's not just about avoiding table salt because of the additives; aside from providing you with sodium, table salt will not do anything else for you. On the other hand, pink Himalayan salt contains sodium chloride as well as 84 different minerals.

It's also natural, and it's thought to have been formed millions of years ago. Two of these minerals include potassium and magnesium, which will help you fight the keto flu.

Not only that, but pink Himalayan salt will help your body better regulate your sleep cycles and blood sugar levels. Don't get me wrong, you can certainly use regular salt on your meals if you prefer the taste of it over other types of salt.

It'll also be more convenient since you likely already have standard table salt at home. However, if you're going to go out of your way and drink salt water to increase your sodium intake, then you might as well use something like pink Himalayan salt or Celtic sea salt.

It'll provide you with more health benefits than something like regular table salt. Of course, salt isn't the only way that you can increase your sodium intake on the dirty keto diet.

You can also use something such as bone broth. Bone broth is essentially bones and connective tissue from animals that's been boiled into a broth and cooked just below boiling point for 10-20 hours.

The broth is also cooked with other things such as herbs and vegetables. Not too long ago, bone broth was something that most people consumed on a daily basis.

Nowadays, most people don't consume bone broth. It has some amazing benefits such as improving skin elasticity and skin moisture, which will help you look younger.

It'll also help with your joint health thanks to the collagen that bone broth contains. It can also help improve your gut health, among many other things.

Potassium

The next electrolyte you're going to want to make sure you get an adequate amount of is potassium. Potassium helps to regulate heart and muscle contractions, and it can also help regulate your blood pressure.

If you have a low amount of potassium, this could be why you experience things such as muscle cramps, muscle twitches, or heart palpitations. When it comes to increasing your potassium intake, what's the first thing most people think of?

Probably a banana right? Well, a banana is high in carbs and that's definitely not something that we're going to want to consume on a dirty keto diet or otherwise.

Therefore, we're going to have to get our potassium from somewhere else; don't worry, we still have some good options. Bananas aren't the only thing that are high in potassium!

As it turns out, avocados are quite high in potassium. In fact, avocados contain around 416 mg of potassium per 3 ounces. Not only that, but avocados are also a good source of healthy fats; they contain a high amount of monounsaturated fat among others.

Since this is a ketogenic diet after all, avocados really are going to be your best friend when you first start out. You'll be able to simultaneously increase your fat intake and your potassium intake by eating one food.

Of course, you're not limited to eating avocados. Greens such as spinach and kale also contain a high amount of potassium.

They contain slightly less potassium per 3 ounces than avocados, but they are still a great source nonetheless. Salmon is another food that can increase your potassium intake, although it does contain the least amount of potassium per 3 ounces at 355 mg.

That's still a good amount though, and salmon will also provide you with a good dose of Omega 3 fatty acids. This will help you improve your ratio of Omega 3's to Omega 6's, which is important since Omega 3 fatty acids act as an anti-inflammatory in the body.

Magnesium

The last electrolyte you're going to want to get an adequate amount of is magnesium. Magnesium has a lot of functions in the body, some of which include preserving muscle and nerve function, supporting the immune system, and maintaining strong bones.

Magnesium is very important for bone health, which most people don't realize. Instead, most people think of calcium when they think of keeping their bones healthy.

Yes, calcium is important for bone health, but calcium can't do its job if proper amounts of magnesium aren't present. Common symptoms you'll want to look out for to see if you have low magnesium are fatigue and muscle weakness, constipation, and an irregular heartbeat.

As far as increasing your magnesium intake is concerned, you have some good options here. The first thing you can do is supplement directly with a magnesium pill. That's an easy way to increase your magnesium intake without having to put any thought into what foods you're eating.

If you want to increase your magnesium intake through your diet, then you still have plenty of keto-friendly options. Various seeds like flax or pumpkin seeds are high in magnesium.

Different kinds of nuts such as almonds are also high in magnesium. Finally, foods such as spinach, mackerel, salmon, and avocados are also high in magnesium.

And as you'll recall, some of these foods (spinach, salmon, and avocados) are also high in potassium, so you can get the most bang for your buck by eating those kinds of foods.

Lastly, you can also supplement directly with electrolytes. Typically, you'll get this in a powder form that you can mix with some water, and you'll be good to go.

Of course, you don't have to supplement with electrolytes if you don't want to. You can easily meet all of your electrolyte needs from dietary food sources alone if you prefer.

Chapter 5: How to Eat Keto at Restaurants, Parties, or Other Social Events

When people start a ketogenic diet, things go well for the first couple of weeks. Then life happens and some sort of event will come up.

Maybe your work decides to cater lunch, you have a wedding to attend, or some other social event is coming up. You tell yourself that you've been following the diet very well for the past couple of weeks, so what could one cheat meal hurt?

You'll get right back on track tomorrow and be back in ketosis before you know it. Next thing you know, tomorrow turns into a week, which turns into a month, and you still haven't gone back to eating keto.

Like I talked about in a previous chapter, it can be hard to get back into keto once you've lost momentum. Don't worry though, in this chapter I'm going to give you some helpful tips and tricks to help you stay on track with your dirty ketogenic diet when you're put in tough situations.

This is the Number One Key for Success on the Dirty Keto Diet

The best thing you can do to ensure success on the dirty keto diet is plan, plan, plan. Being prepared for the given situation is your best line of defense against slipping up on this diet.

What tends to happen on the ketogenic diet is that people get caught in tough, unexpected situations. It can be something like a co-worker bringing cookies to work, or it could something as simple as you being too tired to cook after a long day at work.

These are the types of things that you have to think about in advance. For example, if you know you're going to be too tired to cook after work, then you need to meal prep in advance.

This is critical. It's why I've dedicated an entire chapter to meal prepping; it can make or break your success. In the case of a co-worker bringing cookies to work, you have to remember that you can't eat anything that's high in sugar on this diet plan.

Therefore, if this is something that happens regularly, you need to put a rule into place that says you're not allowed to eat anything high in carbs that your coworkers bring to work.

If that's not good enough and you still find yourself being tempted by peer pressure or something else, then take things one-step further. Set a hard rule in place that states you're not allowed to eat anything your coworkers bring to work. Period.

You only eat the food that you bring to work. This way the decision is made for you in advance, and you don't have to think or worry about it. The same principle of planning in advance will apply to whatever situation you find yourself in.

Sometimes things will come up suddenly, and you'll need to be able to adapt to the given situation. In these instances, you'll have to do your best with what you've got.

However, there are a lot of situations that you'll know are happening in advance. For example, there might be an upcoming party this weekend.

When you find yourself in these types of situations, you must do your best to prepare in advance for what's to come. Here are some helpful tips you can follow that will help you out in various situations you may find yourself in.

What to Do at Parties or Other Social Events

Let's say there's a work Christmas party or some other social event that you know of in advance. What can you do to make sure that you follow your dirty keto diet in these situations?

The first thing you need to do is get in contact with the host. Ask him or her what kinds of food will be at the party. If there are low-carb keto type of foods available, then you know you'll be okay.

If not, then ask if there can be any accommodations made for a low-carb high fat diet that you're currently on. Even if the host isn't able to help you out, there are still a couple of things you can do.

The first would be to ask if it's okay if you bring your own dish to the party. You could explain how you're not the only person at the party who's on a keto diet so other people will enjoy the dish as well.

If that's not an option, there's one of two things you can still do. The first would be to eat a keto meal before you go to the party.

This way you won't be hungry, and you'll be far less tempted to eat something that you shouldn't. The other option you have would be to prepare a keto meal in advance and eat it at the party.

The idea of doing this certainly sounds intimidating. However, if you simply explain to anyone who asks what it is that you're doing, they should be understanding.

Just explain how you're on a keto diet, which is a low-carb and high-fat diet. This is what allows your body to get into ketosis, which is where your body uses fat for fuel instead of carbs.

If you explain this with enthusiasm and passion, you could very well convince other people at the event to start a ketogenic diet! You have to have confidence in what you're doing.

In all actuality, most people won't care what it is that you're eating, or even notice in the first place. If you want proof of this, simply ask yourself if you remember what everyone else ate, drank, and wore to a party that you've been to before.

Chances are good you barely remember any of that stuff! You were probably far more concerned with what *you* were going to eat, drink, and wear to the party.

Once again, you may notice that sticking to your diet plan at parties comes down to planning in advance.

While it may be easier to simply show up to the party and hope that there's something keto approved that you could eat, take the time to plan ahead. Instead of being a victim to the circumstances, you can take matters into your own hands and ensure that you'll be able to stick to your diet plan.

How to Eat Keto at Fast Food Restaurants

Up next we have the common fast food restaurant. Depending on what restaurant you're eating at will determine your game plan, so I want to cover as many different kinds as I can in this section.

The first tip would be to look and see if the place you're eating at has salads on the menu. This can be a great way to consume more greens and eat keto when you're on the go.

However, you have to be careful because not all salads are the same. The main culprit here you need to watch out for is the salad dressing.

Any type of sweet salad dressing such as a raspberry or balsamic vinaigrette will be too high in sugar for you to eat. Ideally, you'll want to add olive oil to the salad that you're eating.

However, any other high-fat dressing such as blue cheese and Caesar dressing would also be acceptable.

Next up are restaurants that serve pizza. This one is tricky because of the crust that contains a lot of carbs. Your best choice would be to eat a cauliflower crust pizza.

This will allow you to eat pizza while avoiding the carbs. However, most pizza places won't serve cauliflower pizza unless it's a specialty restaurant.

Therefore, we're most likely going to have to get creative. The first thing you want to do is load up the pizza with as many keto-approved toppings as possible.

This way you'll be able to fill yourself up on the toppings and not be as tempted to eat something you shouldn't. Next, you want to eat the cheese and toppings on the pizza while avoiding the crust.

This can be hard to do; the best way to go about it would be to use a fork or knife to separate the cheese and toppings from the crust. Finally, you might be able to order thin crust and get away with it depending on how much pizza you plan on eating.

If you're going to do this, make sure that you check the nutrition info first. If the crust contains too many carbs, then you're going to have to pass on it.

In this case, it would simply be better to order a hand tossed pizza. It'll be much easier to separate the cheese and toppings from a hand tossed pizza compared to a thin crust pizza.

Overall though, trying to eat pizza on a ketogenic diet isn't the best idea or the easiest thing to do. If it's possible to eat somewhere else, then you should definitely do that.

However, if you do find yourself at a pizza restaurant, this is the best way to survive while you're following a ketogenic diet.

Up next we have restaurants that serve burgers. This is probably one of the more popular food items you'll see at restaurants in America.

So how can you eat keto at a burger restaurant? The best way to go about things is to order a lettuce wrap.

This is starting to become more and more popular even though a lot of restaurants have yet to catch on. Essentially, the burger is wrapped in lettuce, which is used in place of a bun.

This will help save you on the calories and carbs and allow you to stay in ketosis. As I mentioned before, not all burger places have lettuce wraps, so what should you do in these cases?

Well, the best way to go about things would be to simply pull the bun back slightly and eat the burger in little bites while avoiding the bun. This way you still get the feel of eating a regular burger and the bun will still be able to hold everything in place.

You could also grab a fork and knife and cut up the meat in small pieces and eat that with the toppings in a similar manner to a salad. Now as far as sides are concerned, you're definitely going to have to pass on the fries and soda.

If the restaurant sells a lettuce wrap, then there's a chance that they might have some better side options you can replace the fries with. You might be able to get a side of steamed broccoli or kale chips with your burger instead of fries.

Worst case scenario though, you might not be able to get any sides at all. Even with that being the case, at least it's still possible to eat keto at a burger restaurant.

What about Mexican restaurants? How do you go about eating keto at a Mexican restaurant?

Well as with a lot of things so far, there are some sacrifices that you're going to have to make. However, there are also plenty of good options available to you that'll allow you to still be able to maintain your dirty ketogenic diet.

The first thing that you're going to have to do no matter how difficult is avoid the tortilla chips that are served before your meal. Even if you're eating them with something that contains a low amount of carbs such as guacamole, the chips aren't keto approved; if you eat too many of them, you'll run the risk of getting kicked out of ketosis.

Don't worry, things get much better from here. The first thing you can do is see if you can order your food in a bowl. This is essentially where they take all of the ingredients that they'd normally wrap in a burrito (such as the meat, vegetables, and keto approved sauces that you're adding) and put it into a bowl instead.

61

This is great because it's very similar to what you'd be doing at a burger restaurant except in this case, it'll be much easier to eat. Even if the place you're eating at doesn't offer a bowl option, then you can simply order a burrito with everything you want inside of it.

Then when you get your food, you can unwrap the burrito and eat the contents with a fork. You can do the same thing with fajitas. Simply order the fajitas, but when the food arrives, don't use any of the tortillas that come with the meal.

If you're eating at a place that predominantly sells tacos, you can still do the same thing. You can remove the contents of the taco from the shell and eat them with a fork, almost like you would with a salad.

Your choice of sides may be more limited. Most Mexican restaurants serve rice and beans as their primary sides, and there's usually not much variation to that.

If that's the case, you're definitely going to have to skip out on those sides at the place you're eating at. Instead, see if the restaurant offers the option to double the meats with whatever it is that you're ordering.

If they don't, then your best option would be to order two main courses without the sides or do one main order and load it up with as many vegetables as possible.

Finally, we have Asian restaurants. This is the hardest place to eat at on a keto diet. Things that would normally be keto approved (such as certain meats) aren't in these places because of the way that they're typically prepared.

A lot of the time, these meats will either be breaded or lathered in a sauce that will cause them to contain too many carbs. Cornstarch is another ingredient that's commonly used when preparing Asian dishes, and it's certainly not keto approved.

Therefore, it can be easy to think you're eating keto at an Asian restaurant when in reality, you're not. Additionally, two of the main components of an Asian meal are often going to be fried rice or chow mein.

Neither of these are keto-approved, and that's going to make things a lot more difficult. Another popular side item at Asian restaurants is egg rolls, but again, these aren't keto approved either.

So what can you eat at an Asian restaurant? The first thing would be chicken and broccoli. This is something that a lot of Asian restaurants will have.

The trick is in how it's made. You need to make sure the meat isn't breaded, and you need to ask if it can be served with a keto-approved sauce on the side.

Next up you can see if the place you're eating at serves lettuce wraps. You'll have to double check to see how all of the contents are prepared inside, but it's an option if everything checks out.

And finally we have egg drop soup. Again, this all comes down to how the dish is prepared. Cornstarch is frequently used to make the soup, and it definitely won't be keto if that's the case.

When it comes to eating keto at restaurants, there are some much better options to pick over Asian food. The main reason why people like it in the first place is because of the rice, chow mein, and sauces that are used.

You're not going to be able to eat any of these things on a ketogenic diet anyway, so it's best to avoid Asian restaurants if at all possible. At least in the case of a burger or Mexican restaurant, you're still able to eat the main contents of the meal without any worries about how it was prepared most of the time.

In the case of the Asian restaurant, it's the exact opposite. The dishes will usually be made in a way that doesn't make the food keto-approved anymore.

It's simply best to avoid the temptation altogether in the first place. Once you're in a restaurant and you're ready to order, it can be very hard to leave at that point if they're not going to be able to accommodate to your needs.

This makes it all the more likely that you're going to cheat on your diet plan. You're better off avoiding a sticky situation in the first place if you can help it.

Hopefully these tips gave you some good ideas for how you can eat keto when you're eating at restaurants. Remember, the main thing you want to focus on is being prepared.

That's going to be your best line of defense against eating something that isn't keto approved. Even with that being the case, there will still be times when you're on the go and have to do the best you can with what you've got. That's where these tips will really shine, so be sure to keep them in mind!

Chapter 6: The Importance of Sleep and Why It Can Make or Break Your Success

In this chapter, I'm going to go in depth about why sleep is so important for your fat loss success. You might not think that this is necessary, but it definitely is.

Think about it—you're going to follow this dirty ketogenic diet for a reason right? What is that reason? Are you doing it to feel better and have more energy?

Are you following this keto plan so that you can lose weight? To improve your health? Whatever the reason is, I can assure you that what you eat isn't the only thing that affects your energy levels or your weight.

I don't want this book to be something that simply tells you about the dirty keto diet and then leaves you hoping for the best. I know that there's a certain outcome you want to obtain.

I also know that without a proper mindset or good sleeping habits, you will still fail, even if you follow a great nutrition plan.

In fact, the quantity and quality of your sleep could affect your success more than your diet does. If you're not getting an adequate amount of sleep on a regular basis, then you're going to be fighting an uphill battle in regards to losing weight.

This is because sleep affects key hormones that regulate hunger and how much fat you burn. For this reason, sleep is something you want to take very seriously.

In fact, I'd say sleep is the most important aspect of maintaining a healthy body, followed by your diet, and then exercise. The reason for this is because you're going to spend approximately one-third of your life sleeping.

You'll spend far less time eating and exercising. Therefore, it makes sense to get your sleeping habits in check.

However, most people struggle to get enough sleep at night. We're constantly on the move, always too busy or too stressed out to get a good night's rest; even though it's so important, sleep always seems to take the biggest hit.

We try to make up for the lack of sleep with caffeine, but that can often make things worse depending on when its taken. Before I get into what you need to start doing in order to improve the quality and quantity of your sleep, let's first talk about why sleep is so important to begin with.

Why Sleep Greatly Matters if You Want to Burn Fat

So how much sleep should you be getting on a nightly basis? The research consistently shows that adults need to get around 7-9 hours of sleep per night for optimal health (3).

Even with this being the case, there are still are a lot of people out there who are only getting 6 or even 5 hours of sleep per night. This shouldn't come as a surprise though, as we are busier now more than ever before.

With all of the hustle and bustle that goes on in today's world, something will most likely have to be sacrificed. Hopefully I can make a compelling case for you to prioritize sleep over other things if you're serious about achieving your health and fitness goals.

Firstly, let's focus on how sleep affects your body's ability to burn fat. The first hormones I want to start with are cortisol and melatonin.

You can think of these hormones as opposites in a way. Cortisol signals stress to the body.

If you think about being in fight-or-flight mode, it would be because your body is secreting a high amount of cortisol. When you think of cortisol, you might think of stress and negative things, but cortisol isn't all bad.

The body wouldn't produce something that's purely harmful to itself all of the time. Cortisol is responsible for regulating your body's sleep/wake cycle, your blood sugar levels, and your metabolism.

Cortisol also helps to reduce inflammation. Cortisol creates issues when you produce too much of it at the wrong time, or too much of it too often.

Excessive cortisol levels can cause fatigue, headaches, anxiety, and weight gain, among other things. Ideally, cortisol levels will be at their highest in the morning when you need to wake up and get going for the day.

They should be the lowest when you're trying to go to bed. Melatonin, as I mentioned earlier, can be seen as an opposite to cortisol.

Melatonin helps to regulate sleep/wake cycles by signaling to the body when to relax and rest. Think of melatonin as putting your body in a restful parasympathetic state, whereas cortisol will put your body into a heightened fight-or-flight sympathetic state.

Because of this, it's most ideal to have your melatonin levels be at their highest at night after the sun goes down, and at their lowest in the morning when you're trying to wake up.

Of course, melatonin is responsible for other things, but our primary concern here is how melatonin regulates our sleep cycles. Back in the old days, we would sleep in accordance with the sun.

When the sun rose, we would wake up. When the sun would set, we would go to sleep. This internal and natural cycle that regulates sleepiness and alertness is known as your circadian rhythm or biological clock.

There weren't very many things people could do productivity wise once the sun went down. Nowadays with modern technology, things are much different.

We have artificial light sources that we can use to still get things done during all hours of the day. This might be great for productivity purposes, but it's thrown our hormones and our biological clocks out of whack.

This means that our sleep quality has suffered in recent times. Therefore, the first thing you need to do to improve your sleep quality is to get your biological clock back on track.

The easiest way to do that is to rise with the sun and sleep when the sun sets. Of course, depending on where you live and how much sunlight you get per day, this might not be practical.

The next best thing you could do is sleep during times that are more in accordance with your circadian rhythm. For example, you could go to bed at 10:00 p.m. and wake up at 6:00 a.m.

Or maybe sleeping around 11:00 p.m and waking around 7:00 a.m better fits your schedule. The point is to get to bed earlier and wake up earlier.

Have you ever gone to bed at 2:00 a.m. and woken up at 10:00 a.m. still feeling super tired even though you got eight hours of sleep? I know that I sure have before, but now it makes sense why this happens.

Going to bed at 2:00 a.m. and waking up at 10:00 a.m. completely throws your biological clock out of whack. It causes your body to produce more cortisol at night and less melatonin.

Then you'll be sleeping and your body will be producing less cortisol than it needs to when it's time to wake up. Typically when we stay up late, we're not doing anything productive anyway.

More than likely we're either watching television, or we are on our phones. These electronic devices emit something known as blue light.

Blue light is shorter in wavelength, which causes it to produce more energy. The sun is a producer of blue light, but even after the sun has gone down we can still get exposure to artificial blue light, all thanks to our electronic devices like televisions, cell phones, tablets, and game systems.

The problem with staying on these devices late at night is the fact that blue light exposure will suppress melatonin production because this light spectrum will stimulate alertness. This will not only affect the quality of your sleep, but it will also make it harder for you to fall asleep in the first place.

So what can you do to stop exposure to blue light late at night? The first option you have is to buy some blue light blocking glasses.

These glasses have an orange tint to them, which will help to block the blue light wavelength. Yes, it'll make everything else have a weird coloration to it, but it's worth it if it'll help improve the quality of your sleep.

The cool thing about the glasses is that you can put them on and not have to worry about anything. It doesn't matter if you watch t.v., get on your phone, or play video games—you'll be covered.

Ideally, you'd start to wear these glasses three hours before you go to bed. So if you were going to go to bed at 10:30 p.m., you'd start to wear the glasses at 7:30 p.m.

If the glasses aren't your style, then that's completely fine. Most devices will allow you to download a blue light blocking filter.

For example, you can download an app on your smart phone that will block the blue light that's emitted from your phone. It'll give your phone screen more of an orange tint to it, but it's worth putting up with for the better quality sleep.

The cool thing is that you can set the filter to come on and off at certain times so you don't even have to think about it. The same can also be said for your computer.

You can download a software and have it set to come on at a certain time to block the blue light that's emitted from it. One downside to this is that you may not be able to do this for all of your devices.

Most televisions and video games systems don't have a way for you to be able to block the blue light that comes from them. Sure, you may be covered on some devices such as your smartphone, but if you decide to watch t.v., then you'll still be getting blue light exposure late at night.

That's why I think the glasses are the best way to go. They might not be the most fashionable thing, but most of the time you'll be wearing them late in the day in the comfort of your own home.

You can wear them and forget about the rest regardless of what you're doing. The thing is that blue light can sneak up on us in a lot of different ways that we might not realize.

For instance, the lights you use in your home could stimulate you to stay awake. The glow from your computer or alarm clock could be another culprit.

Or maybe you could look at something on someone else's electronic device and be exposed to blue light in that way. All of these things will affect your body's ability to produce melatonin at night, so you'll want to make sure you avoid blue light during the night as much as you possibly can.

Something you might be thinking of doing right now to get around this would be to take a melatonin supplement. This can be tempting, but I would completely avoid it.

The reason why people commonly take this supplement is because of poor sleep quality. However, when you're taking a melatonin supplement, all you're really doing is addressing a symptom and not the root cause.

For example, you might consistently wake up feeling tired and drowsy and not know why. So you decide to take a melatonin supplement in the hopes that it'll give you better sleep and fix the issue.

It might work for a while, but the real reason that you're waking up tired could be caused by something such as blue light exposure, or you not getting enough sleep at night. These are the real issues that need to be addressed.

You're suppressing your melatonin secretion late at night by being on electronic devices, and then you're trying to make up for it by taking a supplement. This isn't even the main reason why you shouldn't take a melatonin supplement.

The thing is that melatonin is naturally produced by the body. What do you think is going to happen once you start getting your melatonin from an outside source?

Your body will know that you already have plenty of melatonin in your system and that it doesn't need to make any more. Therefore your body will begin to stop the natural production of melatonin.

Not only that, but as times goes on, you'll need to take more and more melatonin in order to get the same effects. When you initially start taking melatonin, you won't need to supplement with that much of it because your body will still be producing high amounts of it.

Over time though, your body will start to decline the amount of melatonin that it's producing. This means that you're going to have to take more melatonin in order to make up for that difference.

Later on down the line, you more than likely won't be able to stop taking melatonin cold turkey. That would completely wreck your sleep cycle. Instead, you'd have to gradually wean yourself off of it in order to signal to your body to start producing melatonin again.

And finally, it's not as if supplements are free. It could cost you quite a bit of money over the long haul if you take a melatonin supplement.

This is why you're better off not taking it in the first place if at all possible. The only exception to this would be if you work a graveyard shift or something similar.

In this case, you're already going to be going against your body's biological clock because you'll be working when you should be naturally sleeping. In this case, taking melatonin will help to put your body in a relaxed and restful state during a time when melatonin production is usually low and cortisol production is higher.

Melatonin and cortisol aren't the only two hormones you need to worry about as far as good sleep is concerned. Not sleeping enough and poor sleep quality affect other hormones as well.

Two big ones are leptin and ghrelin. You can think of these hormones as opposites, similar to melatonin and cortisol.

Leptin is your body's satiety hormone. When leptin is high, it signals to the body that you have enough stored fat and that you don't need to eat any more food.

When leptin is low, this will signal to the body that you don't have enough stored fat and your body will try to conserve energy in an attempt to prevent you from starving to death.

This was great back in the hunter and gatherer days because our ancestors usually didn't know where their next meal was going to come from. Leptin allowed them to hold onto the stored fat that they had in case of an emergency.

In today's world, things are much different. We have food at our fingertips 24/7. We have food in our fridge that we can access anytime time we're at home.

There are plenty of grocery stores and restaurants that are open 24 hours a day. In first world countries, there is no shortage of food.

Regardless of this being the case, our hormones haven't gotten the message. Even if you have plenty of extra stored body fat and plenty of access to food, your body will still act in the same manner.

Your body will want to hold onto that stored fat in case there's a long period of time where you won't have access to food. So if your sleep is out of whack, that's also going to make your leptin levels out of whack.

You definitely don't want your body holding onto your stored fat if it can be prevented in the first place. We also have ghrelin. Like I mentioned earlier, ghrelin acts in a manner opposite to that of leptin.

Ghrelin is your body's hunger hormone. It signals to the body that you're hungry. When you're not feeling hungry, ghrelin levels will be low; when you're feeling, hungry ghrelin levels will be high.

Sleep deprivation will cause an increase in ghrelin and a decrease in leptin. This basically means that you're fighting an uphill battle with your body's hormones.

Under normal circumstances, you might not have these intense feelings of hunger. However, if you're deprived of sleep, then you could be hungry at a time when you normally wouldn't be.

In addition to that, lack of sleep will also affect your willpower. Imagine for instance that you get plenty of sleep.

You wake up feeling good about yourself, you exercise for a bit, and eat a healthy breakfast. How likely do you think it is that you're going to eat a good keto meal for lunch and dinner that day?

How likely is it that you'll be able to avoid tempting foods that your coworkers may bring to work? The answer to that is pretty darn likely.

You're feeling good about yourself, and you've been able to build momentum at the very start of your day. This is all because you got plenty of sleep at night and you're now able to make better decisions as the day goes on.

Now compare that scenario to something much different. Let's say this time you don't get a good night's sleep.

Maybe there was something really stressful at work or something came up with your family which caused you to only get 5 hours of sleep that night. What do you think is going to happen the next day?

Well, more than likely you're going to wake up feeling rushed because you'll want to sleep in for as long as possible. You hit the snooze button a few times before getting up.

Then once you did get up, you found yourself rushing to get to work on time. You didn't have any time to eat a healthy breakfast or exercise before work.

Then once you're at work, you're probably going to feel hungrier and more irritable than you usually do thanks to the increased ghrelin. Now when your coworker brings cookies for everyone to eat at lunch, you're far more likely to indulge.

You might find yourself already eating the cookie before you even realize what's going on. Then once you realize how eating this cookie goes against your diet plan, you'll start to feel guilty about yourself and tailspin out of control, possibly taking weeks before you get things back on track.

And this was all because your sleep got thrown off the night before. A lot of times when it comes to dieting, people only tend to think about the mechanical part of the process.

For example, people think about what they need to eat, what they need to avoid, and if they stick to that, they will be good to go. What people often fail to think about is how we're making the decisions that we are.

For instance, someone might think that he or she is bad at following a diet plan because of consistently failing to be able to stick to anything. The truth is that it could all be because of some other factor; Perhaps a poor self-image or lack of sleep is holding the person back from making the correct decision.

Hopefully you now see the importance of getting enough quality sleep at night. Now the question becomes what you can do to improve your sleep quality and quantity at night.

How to Improve Your Sleep Quality and Quantity at Night

Getting enough sleep is a big factor in the equation of our health and fat loss journey. Even if you're getting 4 hours of quality sleep each and every night, that won't be long enough for you to get the full benefits of sleep.

You need to make sure that you're falling into that 7-9 hour range that we talked about earlier. One of the main reasons for this is because our body sleeps in cycles.

There are 5 different stages of sleep. The first stage is a light sleep, and the second stage prepares the body for the deep sleep that comes during stages 3 and 4. The last stage is rapid eye movement sleep (REM).

During the final stage of REM sleep, the eyes are still closed, but your eyes are rapidly moving as the name implies. Each sleep cycle will typically take around 90 minutes or so.

Ideally, you'd want to wake up at the completion of a sleep cycle. For you, this could mean getting 7.5 hours of sleep per night or even 9. It really depends though, as some sleep cycles are slightly longer than 90 minutes; if that's the case, 8 hours of sleep might be right for you.

You'll have to test it out and see what works best for you. And if you've ever gotten plenty of sleep, yet you still woke up tired, then it could be because you woke up during a deep stage of sleep such as stage 3 or 4.

If you're only getting 5 hours of sleep per night for instance, then you're not giving your body much of a chance to complete the correct number of sleep cycles that it needs to. Not only is sleep important for fat loss purposes, but you also need sleep for other things.

Sleep helps your immune system function properly. It's definitely going to be harder to reach your fitness goals if you're regularly getting sick.

And sleep is also important for memory consolidation. If you're sleep deprived, then you'll have a harder time retaining information compared to someone who's getting an adequate amount of sleep each night.

Now let's talk about what you can do to increase the amount of time that you're sleeping each night if you're currently struggling with that. The first tip would be to see what time you're usually going to bed at night.

If you need to get more sleep at night, the first solution is to start going to bed earlier, although this is typically easier said than done. Usually, this is where the problem lies; you have to get up early for work, but you're going to bed too late.

See when it is that you're generally going to bed, and notice what you are doing late at night. Are you using the electronic devices that are stimulating you to stay awake?

Maybe you're eating foods late at night that are causing you to stay up. Whatever it is, you need to become aware of it so you can fix the problem.

For example, it's going to be hard to go to bed earlier if you're on your phone late at night. Therefore, the first thing that you must do is cut out distractions late at night.

You don't want to be doing anything that can stimulate you to stay up later than you're supposed to. Even if you're using blue-light blocking glasses, things such as social media on your phone can be easy to scroll through endlessly; next thing you know, it's suddenly an hour past your bedtime.

That's why you're better off following the rule of no electronic devices an hour before bedtime. This will make things much easier for you to be able to get to bed on time.

When I was trying to get a consistent sleep schedule down, I really struggled. Eventually I realized that I struggled because I kept watching videos on my phone late at night. One video would lead to the next and before I knew it, it was 2 a.m.

Even with the blue light filter on, it didn't matter. My phone was distracting me from getting to bed on time.

My solution to this problem was to set an alarm for when it was time for me to start getting ready to go to bed. Most people only set alarms for when it's time to wake up, but why not set an alarm to alert you when it's time to go to bed as well?

I go to bed around 10:30 p.m. every night, so I set an alarm for 9:30 p.m. This tells me to stop the use of all electronic devices and to start getting ready for bed.

My phone even has a feature that'll lock me out of any potentially distracting apps. After you do that, you'll definitely want to make sure that you go to bed and wake up at the same time every day of the week.

This is actually the most important tip for improving your sleep quality and energy levels. Think about what it is that most people do.

They'll wake up at the same time 5 days per week to go to work, but they will sleep in during the weekend. You're not giving your body a consistent schedule to adapt to when you do that.

Your body starts to adjust to waking up around 7:00 a.m. every day. Then the weekend comes around and you sleep in until 10:30 a.m, and suddenly your body is confused. When Monday comes around, your body will be stuck trying to wake up at 10:30 a.m instead of 7:00 a.m.

Your body won't know what to think. You'll likely wake up a little tired on Monday because you're trying to get back into the swing of things.

You probably won't get back on track until Wednesday, but by Friday night you'll throw things all out of whack again. The only solution to this is to wake up at the same time every single day of the week.

A more structured sleep will allow your body to know when it's time to start producing melatonin at night and when it's time to start producing cortisol in the morning. I know you might be turned off to the idea of this, but I promise it works.

Before I did this, I was always tired and frequently took naps. Now I wake up feeling well rested, and I feel energized throughout the day.

Of course, you might be wondering, what am I supposed to do on the weekends when I wake up early? Well, there are plenty of things to do!

You could do something relaxing such as reading a book. You could exercise, or you could start your meal prepping for the week.

The point is that you want to find something, and it needs to be important. Personally, if what I'm doing in the morning isn't that important to me, then I'm far more likely to sleep in.

I'm willing to bet that you might be the same way. If reading a book doesn't sound that appealing to you at 7:00 a.m. on a Saturday morning, then you'll need to find something else.

Meal prepping is a really solid option to do during this time. It's important, and it'll help set you up for a good week on the keto diet plan.

You'll get it out of the way first thing in the morning, and you'll have time during the rest of the day to do whatever it is that you want. You could even split up your meal prepping during Saturday and Sunday mornings so that you have something to do on both days.

If you did this, you'd set yourself up for major success on the ketogenic diet. Of course, meal prepping isn't your only option.

You just need to find something you're interested in doing during your weekend mornings. If you find yourself struggling to get started with this tip, there are a couple of things that you can do.

The first thing is to make sure that you set your alarm clock across the room from where you sleep before you go to bed. For example, if you use your phone as an alarm clock, then set it across the room so that you have to get out of your bed in order to turn it off in the morning.

This will also help prevent you from staying on your phone late at night. If it's within arms reach, then it's far too easy to turn the alarm off and go back to bed.

This is a simple tip but it works wonders. Now you might be thinking, "Thomas, I've tried that before and it didn't work!" Perhaps you would just get up, turn off my alarm, and then go right back to bed.

If this is the case, you'll need to get more creative. For example, you might need to buy a special light that can be controlled through an app on your phone. These light bulbs aren't that expensive either (usually $20 or less) and you can program the light to come on during a certain time of the day.

If you're trying to get up at 7:00 a.m., then you could set the light to come on at 7:00 a.m. and have your alarm go off at that time as well. If that's still not enough, then get multiple alarm clocks and set them up in opposite corners in your room.

Then when all of them go off at once, it'll be really loud and you'll be wide awake by the time you turn all of them off. Secondly, get excited the night before, as if you have something to really look forward to in the morning.

Think about a kid on Christmas morning. Are they thinking negative thoughts before going to bed that night? No, of course not!

They're full of energy and ready to go at 5 or 6 in the morning because they can't wait to open presents! However, as adults, we typically think about how we aren't going to get a lot of sleep after getting home late, or how tired we will be in the morning after only sleeping a few hours.

Instead of thinking thoughts about how tired we're going to be in the morning, why not think in the opposite manner?

Think about things such as, "I'm getting plenty of sleep tonight. I'm going to wake up tomorrow fully rested and full of energy!" You'll want to do this regardless of how much sleep it is that you're going to be getting that night.

While you ideally want to get 7-9 hours of sleep per night, there will still be some nights where you don't hit that number. These are the nights when thinking positive thoughts before bed will come in handy.

You can even go as far as practicing waking up excited during the middle of the day. I've done this before, and it works really well. Simply set your alarm for one minute past the current time and then when it goes off, spring out of bed with excitement.

By doing this, you're starting to train your brain to view your alarm as a positive thing, not a negative thing. If you currently view your alarm ringtone as negative, then change it to something else.

This way you can start to associate that ring with positive feelings and thoughts rather than negative ones. The main thing is to be creative and not make excuses; this tip of waking up at the same time every day can make or break your success.

Now let's get into some more specific tips you can do to improve your sleep quality at night. A lot of these tips work hand-in-hand with each other as far as sleep quality and quantity is concerned.

For example, drinking caffeine late at night will affect both your sleep quality and quantity. Caffeine is a good place to start.

You definitely don't want to consume any caffeine at least 10 hours before you go to bed. For example, if you're going to bed at 11:00 p.m., then you don't want to consume any caffeine past 1:00 p.m.

It might not sound too harmful to drink coffee later than that, but the thing most people don't realize is that caffeine stays in your system for hours after you drink it. Therefore, that coffee you had in the late afternoon could be affecting your sleep later that night.

Some people might try to mask this issue by taking melatonin, but the better thing to do would be to stop drinking coffee so late in the day. If you're drinking coffee that late to become more alert, then there's something deeper with your sleep that needs to be fixed Drinking more coffee isn't the solution.

Another thing you'll want to avoid doing is drinking alcohol late at night. This is a keto diet so most alcohol isn't keto-approved anyway, however, you do still have some options that I'll cover later on.

For now though, understand that alcohol and the quality of your sleep don't go hand-in-hand. Sure, drinking some alcohol might put your body in a relaxed state and make it easier for you to fall asleep, but you'll pay the price during the night.

Alcohol affects your REM sleep, which can cause you to wake up in the middle of the night, snore, and sleepwalk during the night. When you wake up, you might feel groggy and irritable.

Aside from avoiding alcohol and caffeine, something you can do to help you fall asleep faster is to start a journal. No, I'm not talking about keeping a journal like a teenager going through a breakup.

Instead, we're going to use this journal to help get all of our thoughts down on paper before bedtime. Whenever you try to go to sleep, have you ever noticed how your mind is racing with thoughts?

You could spend 30 minutes just thinking of different things about your day before you're able to actually fall asleep. Well, journaling at night before you go to bed will help with that.

Just do a complete brain dump of anything you're thinking about and write it down. Don't even think, just keep writing for 5 minutes straight and get everything down on the paper.

Then when it's time to go to bed, you should notice that your mind is a lot calmer and that it's much easier to fall asleep. There's something special about putting your thoughts down on paper that helps calm down our brain.

These final two tips might not seem that important, but they can make a big difference. The first one is to make sure that you're clean before you go to bed. Research shows that we sleep better at night when we're clean (4). This means that you need to take a shower at night before going to bed in order to improve your sleep quality.

I understand that a lot of people might take a shower in the morning. The shower might be used as a way to wake up and get their morning started.

However, if you think about it, it makes more sense to take a shower before bed. This way you won't go to sleep at night feeling dirty or smelly, which will help improve the quality of your sleep at night.

Not only that, but if you're taking showers in the morning as a way to help wake yourself, you'll no longer need to do that if you're following the other tips I've talked about. Finally, the last thing you need to do in order to improve your sleep quality is to make your bedroom as dark as possible when you're going to bed.

You don't want any light coming from computer screens, televisions, alarm clocks, or night lights in your room. The reason for this is because these blue lights will affect your body's ability to produce melatonin at night. This will obviously impact the quality of your sleep.

If implementing all of these tips at once sounds overwhelming to you, then only start with a few of them. Try out the ones you think will have the biggest impact on your sleep and then go from there.

For instance, you could start by placing your phone across the room when you sleep and avoiding electronic devices for at least an hour before you go to bed. After you've gotten those habits down, you can move onto something else such as waking up at the same time every day of the week.

The best thing you can do in regards to your sleep is to take action on some or all of these habits now. Don't delay. I know first hand how easy it can be to put off better sleep habits until the next night, and trust me it's not worth it.

Chapter 7: How to Meal Prep on a Ketogenic Diet

Meal prepping is the single most important thing that you can do in order to drastically increase your chances of success on the dirty ketogenic diet. The reason for this is because you failing to prepare is setting you up to fail.

Meal prepping essentially takes all of the decisions and work you'd have to do during the week and condenses it down into one or two days. A lot of this has to do with decision fatigue as I talked about in an earlier chapter.

This is something most people don't know about, and therefore it's not a threat they see coming that can ruin their success. For example, if you're eating 3 meals a day each day of the week, then that's a total of 21 meals per week.

For most people, this would mean that they're making 21 individual decisions about what they want to eat. Then they have to get the necessary ingredients to make whatever meal it is they want to eat. After that, they have to prepare the meal, eat it, and then clean up afterwards.

That's a lot of decisions and things that you're going to have to do in order to eat properly on this keto diet. That might not seem like a big deal as you're reading this. However, you can't think of things in the present moment when you're feeling good.

Imagine yourself after a long day at work. If you have children, you have to come home and take care of them. Are you going to feel like cooking and preparing a ketogenic meal 100% of the time in these situations?

For most people, the answer is probably no. And when you are on the ketogenic diet, all it takes is one mess up before you could potentially be on a slippery slope; it might take days or even weeks before you get back on track.

It's best to think of these things that might derail you from success in advance and plan for them ahead of time. That's essentially what the goal of meal prepping is, which is why it's so critical to your success on this diet plan in particular.

If you were following a different diet plan, maybe one that wasn't strict on how much protein, carbs, and fat you needed to eat, then meal prepping wouldn't matter as much. For example, let's say you're following a particular style of the 'if it fits your macros' diet that allows you to eat any foods you want as long as it fits within your macro percentages for the day.

And just so we're clear, I don't recommend following this style of the 'if it fits your macros' diet. However, for the sake of example, if you were following this diet plan, then meal prepping wouldn't be nearly as critical as it is on the ketogenic diet.

The reason for this is because you could easily eat fast food or processed foods quite often and still be on track with your diet plan. But in terms of the ketogenic diet, meal prepping will not only help to increase your chances of success on the diet, but it'll also help you save a lot of time.

By cooking in batches, you'll be saving time setting up to cook, and you'll also have fewer dishes to clean. Meal prepping can also save you money because you'll prepare the exact amount of food that you'll need to eat. you won't have to worry about wasting any of the excess.

Now that we've talked about some of the benefits to meal prepping, let's get into the actual process of how to go about doing it.

The Step-By-Step Process to Successfully Meal Prep on the Dirty Keto Diet

Here's the exact step-by-step process you need to follow in order to see success in regards to meal prepping on the ketogenic diet.

Step #1: Decide when it is that you want to meal prep

The first thing that you need to do is figure out when you want to meal prep. For most people, the best time to do this would be on a Sunday afternoon.

Usually, these days are going to be pretty relaxing and chill. You might not be doing anything on these days aside from watching sports, so you might as well prepare for the upcoming week while the games are on.

Of course, you're not limited to doing this on just Sundays. Depending on what your schedule is, a different day of the week might work better for you. The point is to try and meal prep on a day when you're off from work and you don't have much else going on.

If you don't want to meal prep on a single day, you can always split it up between two days. For example, on Sunday you could prep all of your meals for Monday, Tuesday, and Wednesday.

Then on Wednesday, you could prep your meals for the rest of the week. Be honest with yourself about how likely it is that you're going to stick to this regime.

If you're working a 9-to-5 job Monday through Friday, this would mean that you're going to have to plan and prepare for the rest of your meals on a day when you have to work.

If going to work gives you momentum to continue doing something productive for the rest of the day, then this could be a great option for you. However, if you know that you're likely not going to feel like doing much after work, then it's best to do all of your meal prepping on a single day when you're off from work.

I wouldn't recommend splitting up your meal prepping across more than two days. Anything more than that and it defeats the purpose of what we're trying to achieve in the first place.

Finally, you could meal prep during the mornings on the weekend if you're going to be waking up at the same time every day like I talked about in the chapter on sleep.

This would be a great way to maintain your new sleep schedule because you'd have something to do when you wake up. There's not a right or wrong time to choose when it comes to doing your meal prep. The main thing is that you're able to consistently do it, so pick a time when you're most likely to get the job done.

Step #2: Plan out all of your meals

This could be one of the more difficult steps in the process, however, it will get easier as time goes on. You'll be eating similar meals, and you'll know exactly what you need to buy and how to make it.

Initially, this can be a bit tedious. Remember though, this is something you would have to think about multiple times a day, and you'd have to make these decisions when you're mentally drained.

At least this way, you're fresh and you'll have an easier time making the correct decisions. The easiest way to go about doing this would be to use pen and paper or a spreadsheet.

You would write breakfast, lunch, and dinner going across the top row of the spreadsheet, and then you would write the days of the week going down the first column.

From here, you have a couple of different options as to what you can do. You can plan out all of your breakfasts for the week, then all of your lunches, followed by all of your dinners.

Or you can plan out all of your meals for Monday, then Tuesday, etc. Don't feel as if you need to eat 21 different meals over the course of the week. Keep things as simple as possible.

Initially, you might only want to try eating 2-3 different meals for breakfast as well as for lunch and dinner. For example, for breakfast, you might eat eggs and bacon on Monday. Then on Tuesday, you might make a cheddar cheese omelet.

And you'd simply rotate between eating these two breakfast meals throughout the week. This way you won't stress yourself out trying to think of different meals to eat.

And whether you are aware of this or not, people typically eat the same things more often than they realize. As time goes on, you can try out different meals; you're certainly not limited to the meals you can eat as long as they're keto approved.

Step #3: Work Out Your Macro Percentages

Steps 3 and 4 are interchangeable. You can do whichever one you prefer first. The benefit of calculating your macro percentages first is that you'll know exactly how much food you need to get at the grocery store.

On the other hand, if you go to the grocery store first, then you'll be estimating how much of certain foods you'll need. This, of course, isn't that big of a deal because if you're unsure, you can always buy more than you think you need. This would give you some leftovers for the following week.

Essentially though, what you need to do for this step is to figure out how much of each meal you're going to eat. Let's use the example of eating bacon and eggs for breakfast on Monday.

During this step, you need to figure out how many eggs it is that you're going to eat. Let's say you decide to eat 3 eggs. How are they going to be prepared? How much bacon are you going to eat?

These factors will affect the total caloric content and the macros. This is why it's a good idea to know ahead of time roughly how many calories it is that you want to consume per meal.

For example, if you're eating 2,000 calories a day, how do you want to break that up across your meals? You could do an even split between breakfast, lunch, and dinner, but you don't have to do that if you don't want to.

Some people (such as myself) prefer to eat smaller breakfasts and larger dinners. The reason why I personally like doing this is because breakfast isn't that social of a meal.

You're typically eating breakfast by yourself. With dinner though, you'll usually be eating that meal with friends or family, and it's more enjoyable if you can eat more calories.

If breakfast is an important meal in your household, you could always eat a large breakfast and a smaller dinner. It doesn't matter how you want to break up your calories across your meals. Simply do whatever will work best for you.

Once you've decided how many calories it is that you want to eat for each meal, you'll then have the framework you need to determine how much of certain foods you'll need to eat. Continuing on with our example of eating 2,000 calories per day, let's say the individual decides to split up his calories evenly across 3 meals.

This would mean that he's going to eat 667 calories per meal. In the case of eating bacon and eggs for breakfast, he could eat 4 fried eggs and 6 slices of bacon, assuming that each fried egg contains around 90 calories and each slice of bacon contains around 50 calories.

From here, all he would have to do is track how much fat and protein is contained in the eggs and bacon and he'd be good to go for this meal. Then on Tuesday, let's say he wants to eat the cheddar cheese omelet, and it's going to require 6 eggs to make.

If he's rotating between these two breakfast meals, then he knows that he'll need to get three dozen eggs to meal prep his breakfasts when he goes to the store to shop for his weekly groceries.

You would then repeat this process for lunch and dinner. After completing this process, you'd know exactly what it is that you need to get at the grocery store, which is why I recommend doing this step first before you buy your groceries.

Step #4: Buy your groceries

After you've determined what meals you're going to eat and how much of each food item you need, the next thing you need to do is go grocery shopping. If you're following things in the order I've outlined, all of the legwork has been done upfront.

Depending on what you're shopping for, you can buy in bulk or on a week to week basis. For example, different kinds of nuts you'll be eating on this dirty keto diet have long expiration dates.

You could buy these types of food items in bulk so that you always have some on hand, and you might be able to get a discount on them. However, most of the things you'll be buying will have short expiration dates.

This would include various things such as vegetables or dairy products. You're more than likely going to be better off buying these things on a week-to-week basis.

Buying in bulk when you can is great because it'll be that much less you have to shop for the following week. At the end of the day, shop in a manner that's easiest for you.

If grocery shopping once a week and getting the same things every time keeps things simple for you, then by all means do it. On the flip side, if you like buying in bulk, then do that whenever possible.

Step #5: Cook Your Meals

Now it's time for the fun part. You're going to cook and prepare your meals ahead of time. This will take a good chunk of your time, but there are some things you can do to save some time.

The first thing would be to start cooking the foods that will take the longest. For example, if there's some meat that needs to be slow-cooked, then go ahead and get that started first.

You can start preparing and cooking other things after you get that going. This'll help save you a lot of time because you don't want to wait until the end to start cooking something that's going to take 6 hours to finish.

The next tip is to cook in batches of individual ingredients when possible. For example, let's say one of your lunches is going to consist of a chicken salad with steamed broccoli, cheese, and olive oil for the dressing.

You don't have to prepare the broccoli and chicken in the same skillet. Instead, it's much easier to prepare all of the chicken that you're going to need for the week.

After you start preparing the chicken, you can separately prepare the other ingredients such as broccoli. Then once you're done, you'll be able to put the ingredients together for certain meals as needed.

Of course, this might not be possible for all of your meals. With certain meals on your calendar, you might not be able to add in ingredients later on. In these cases, go ahead and make everything together at once.

However, if you want to save some time, cook everything separately first and then combine ingredients later on whenever possible. The final tip is to be organized and have a plan ahead of time.

Know what it is that you need to get cooked and know the best order to cook it in. Whenever you have something baking in the oven, use that time to start cutting up vegetables or something else.

The better your plan of action, the smoother things will go. Know exactly what utensils, spices, oils, and other things you'll need and have them ready to go before you start. This can save you some time by preventing you from scrambling when you need something.

Step #6: Put Your Meals in Containers and Store Them

At this point, pat yourself on the back because most of the hard work has been done. Once everything has been cooked, you'll simply need to put all of your meals into meal prep containers and store them in a refrigerator.

As far as what kind of containers you should get, I recommend getting some nice glass meal prep containers. With glass containers, you don't have to worry about them containing any BPA's, and you won't have to worry about them not being microwave or dishwasher safe.

Of course, if you fear you might drop your containers, plastic isn't a bad option. Make sure you invest in some high-quality containers. You want these containers to last for a long time to come.

As long as the plastic containers are BPA free and microwave and dishwasher safe, then you'll be good to go. Some of the containers might even have separated compartments within them.

This is certainly handy depending on what meal you're eating, but it isn't necessary. Just go with whatever suits your particular needs best!

Finally, the last thing you'll want to make sure you do is label your containers. You don't want to have to look around and hunt down what you're going to eat for the day.

A simple label saying something like, "Monday's Breakfast", will easily suffice. This will help save you a lot of time.

The last thing you want is to be rushed in the morning and accidentally grab the wrong container before you head off to work. Labeling the containers will keep things clean and organized.

And as a side note, if you don't have enough room in your main refrigerator for all of these containers, then consider buying a mini fridge to store some or all of your prepped meals.

This is a great option if you have a family. You'll only have to worry about eating from your own fridge.

You won't be tempted by anything that's in the main fridge if your spouse isn't following a ketogenic diet. Hopefully you won't have to worry as much about your kids getting into your prepped meals either.

All in all though, make sure that you prepare in advance as much as you possibly can. Sticking to this diet plan isn't about having a lot of willpower, it's more about being prepared. If you can do that, then you'll be setting yourself up for a much greater chance of success.

Chapter 8: Building Muscle on a Dirty Ketogenic Diet

Throughout this book, I've talked about using the dirty ketogenic diet strictly for weight loss purposes. The majority of the people who are interested in the ketogenic diet want to follow it to lose weight.

However, your fitness goal may be different. You might be interested in building muscle, or maybe you want to lose some fat now and add some muscle down the line.

In this chapter, you're going to learn everything you need to know about building muscle on a ketogenic diet.

How Do Things Change When You Want to Build Muscle?

When you're trying to lose weight, the goal is to create a caloric deficit by burning off more calories than you consume. However, when you're trying to build muscle, you want to do the opposite.

You want to create a caloric surplus by eating more calories than you burn off. The reason for this is because you need to give your body enough of the raw materials it needs in order to pack on some new muscle.

Think of it like building a house. Let's say for the sake of example that you need 10,000 bricks to build a certain size house.

If your brick supplier is only able to supply you with 8,000 bricks, then the max-sized house you're going to be able to build is going to be smaller than you originally hoped for.

The same is true for your body. If your body needs 2,800 calories a day in order to maximize muscle gains, then if you don't eat that many calories you're going to be leaving muscle on the table.

Nutritionally, the amount of calories that you eat is the biggest difference between building muscle and burning fat. The other big difference between burning fat and building muscle is how you exercise.

If you're trying to burn fat, then you don't have to exercise at all if you don't want to. You can lose weight solely by following your diet plan.

Conversely, when it comes to building muscle you're going to need to do some form of resistance training. The reason for this is because you must provide your body with some sort of stimulus in order to build muscle.

If you're sedentary and eat more calories than you burn off, you'll just gain fat. Therefore, by working out, you'll be providing your body with a reason to grow back bigger and stronger.

Then once you combine working out with the right nutrition plan, you will start to build muscle. If you're interested in building muscle, the only thing that's going to change with the dirty keto diet is the total amount of calories that you're eating.

Everything else stays the same. Your macro percentages are the same, and the guidelines of what you can and can't eat stay the same, as well as everything else. The question now becomes how much you should eat in order to start building muscle.

How Many Calories Should You Eat to Build Muscle?

If you'll recall from an earlier chapter, we determined our resting metabolic rate which is the total number of calories someone burns per day by taking our current bodyweight and multiplying it by 13.

We're going to have the same starting point as if we're trying to burn fat. The difference is where we're going from that starting point.

Let's use an example of someone who currently weighs 200 pounds. He would take 200 and multiply that by 13 to get a total of 2,600.

This means that this individual burns off 2,600 calories in a given day. If he wanted to start losing weight he would need to eat less than this number.

However, if he wants to start building muscle, then he needs to eat more than this. The trick is to not eat way above this number.

The reason for this is because eating too many calories can lead to excess fat gain. We essentially want to eat enough to build muscle, but not too much to the point where we gain fat.

The best way to strike this balance is to aim to gain half a pound a week. This means that you'll need to add 250 calories to your resting metabolic rate because it takes a surplus of roughly 3,500 calories to gain one pound.

Continuing on with our example, this person would take his resting metabolic rate of 2,600 and add 250 to it to get a total of 2,850.

Therefore, this person would need to eat 2,850 calories per day in order to gain half a pound of muscle per week. Once this step is done, the next thing you need to do is calculate your macro percentages.

As I mentioned earlier, the percentages of fat, protein, and carbs that you're going to eat stay the same, regardless of whether the goal is to build muscle or to burn fat.

This means we're still going to eat 75% of our total calories from fat, 20% from protein, and the remaining 5% from carbs. Here's a breakdown of what that looks like:

2,850 x 0.75= 2,137.5 calories per day from fat
2,850 x 0.2= 570 calories per day from protein
2,850 x 0.05= 142.5 calories per day from carbs

We can then determine the gram equivalent by doing the following:

2,137.5/9 = 237.5 grams of fat per day
570/4 = 142.5 grams of protein per day
142.5/4 = 35.6 grams of carbs per day

From here all you have to do is stay on track with your calories and macros, and you'll be good to go. You don't have to worry about changing any of the fundamentals of the dirty keto diet when your primary goal is to build muscle.

Workout You Can Use to Build Muscle

The last thing I want to leave you with before I wrap up this chapter is a muscle-building workout that you can do at the gym. It's a very simple routine, but that doesn't mean it's ineffective.

As long as you focus on increasing the amount of weight you lift over time, then you'll be good to go. Here's the workout:

Monday: Push Workout

- Incline Dumbbell Bench Press—3 sets of 6 reps, 2 minutes rest between sets
- Standing Dumbbell Military Press—3 sets of 8 reps, 90 seconds rest between sets
- Standing Dumbbell Lateral Raises—3 sets of 10 reps, 60 seconds rest between sets
- Tricep Rope Pushdowns—3 sets of 12 reps, 60 seconds rest between sets
- Tricep Dumbbell Kickbacks—3 sets of 12 reps, 60 seconds rest between sets

Wednesday: Pull Workout

- Lat Pulldowns—3 sets of 8 reps, 90 seconds rest between sets
- Chest Supported Dumbbell Row—3 sets of 8 reps, 90 seconds rest between sets
- Bent Over Flys with Dumbbells—3 sets of 12 reps, 60 seconds rest between sets
- Standing Barbell Curls—3 sets of 8 reps, 90 seconds rest between sets
- Incline Dumbbell Curls—3 sets of 10 reps, 60 seconds rest between sets

Friday: Leg Workout

- Goblet Squats—3 sets of 8 reps, 90 seconds rest between sets

- Leg Press—3 sets of 8 reps, 90 seconds rest between sets
- Leg Extensions—3 sets of 10 reps, 60 seconds rest between sets
- Hamstring Curls—3 sets of 10 reps, 60 seconds rest between sets
- Standing Calf Raises—3 sets of 15 reps, 45 seconds rest between sets

Note: A rep is one complete motion of an exercise and a set is a series of repetitions. For example, on the standing barbell curl exercise, you're doing the movement for 3 sets of 8 reps per set.

One single rep of the exercise would be you curling the bar upwards from resting on your thighs towards your shoulders. Then you would control the bar on the way back down to the starting position.

Once the barbell returns to the starting position, that completes one rep. You'd complete that movement 7 more times for a total of 8 reps.

Once you reach 8 reps, you would then take the prescribed amount of rest time, which in this case is 90 seconds. After the rest period is up, you would then perform another 8 reps, which would complete set number 2.

You would rest another 90 seconds before completing your final set consisting of 8 repetitions. After the third set, you would then move on and start the next exercise.

Chapter 9: Frequently Asked Questions

What Kinds of Foods Should I Eat on a Dirty Ketogenic Diet?

You might be wondering what some good food choices are for this diet plan. Here are some good ideas for fat, protein, and carb sources:

Protein:

- Lean meats such as chicken, beef, venison, turkey, etc.
- Fish
- Eggs
- Cottage cheese

Fat:

- Eggs
- Avocados
- Olive and coconut oil
- Flax and chia seeds
- Various nuts such as pecans and macadamia nuts
- Cheese

Carbs:

- Kale
- Spinach
- Broccoli
- Cauliflower

- Berries such as raspberries and blackberries due to their low net carbs. (Always be sure to check that they fit within your macros.)

Spices:

- Rosemary
- Pink Himalayan salt
- Black pepper
- Oregano
- Basil

This isn't a comprehensive list by any means. These are just some ideas to get you started. As long as you're eating a high amount of fat, a moderate amount of protein, and a low amount of carbs, then you'll be good to go.

What Are Some Popular Foods People Think Are Keto Approved But Aren't?

This is definitely something you want to think about before you start the dirty keto plan. You don't want to regularly eat something you think is keto approved when in reality, it isn't. Here are some popular foods people think are okay to eat on a keto diet, but aren't in reality:

Carrots: you might think that carrots are okay to eat on a ketogenic diet because they're a vegetable, and vegetables are good for you. While that certainly is the case, that doesn't mean that all vegetables are acceptable on certain diet plans.

The reality is that carrots contain too much sugar and have too many net carbs for them to be acceptable on this diet plan. Most leafy green vegetables contain a lot of fiber, making their net carbs zero or very close to it.

This allows you to eat as many of these kinds of vegetables as you please and not have the worry about getting kicked out of ketosis. The same can't be said for carrots, so it's best to avoid them altogether.

Fruit: this can be another tricky food item for some people to wrap their mind around as to why it's not okay to eat. Our whole lives, we've been told that fruit is good for us due to the rich amount of vitamins and nutrients that they contain.

While this may be true, that doesn't mean that fruit is good for you on certain diet plans. On the dirty ketogenic diet plan, fruit isn't going to do you any favors.

It contains a high amount of fructose, which will kick you out of ketosis. The only real exception to this are raspberries and blackberries.

These berries specifically contain a low enough amount of net carbs that you can enjoy some from time to time and not have to worry about getting kicked out of ketosis.

Certain Nuts Such as Cashews and Walnuts: Not all nuts are keto approved, and the main reason for this is because some nuts contain a high amount of net carbs. Cashews are the worst nut that you can eat on a ketogenic diet because they contain the highest amount of net carbs.

Walnuts also contain a good amount of net carbs, although it's not quite as high as cashews. Almonds could also be included on this list, even though they are low enough in net carbs for you to be able to enjoy some from time to time.

Almonds are probably one of the most popular nuts that exist, but they're overrated, especially on a ketogenic diet. They contain a higher amount of net carbs than other nuts, and they contain a high amount of Omega 6 fatty acids.

This type of fat acts as in inflammatory in the body, and most people need to improve the ratio of Omega 3's (which acts as an anti-inflammatory) to Omega 6's in their diet.

Almonds simply won't help you out in that regard. However, the overall amount of net carbs is low enough to where you could have some here and there if you really wanted to. At the end of the day though, there are simply some better choices out there when it comes to nuts.

Am I Allowed to Drink Alcohol on the Dirty Ketogenic Diet?

For the most part, you're going to be very limited on what you can have as far as alcohol is concerned on the ketogenic diet. Most beers are going to contain too many carbs, which will kick you out of ketosis.

However, there are some light beers that you could have. You'll definitely want to check and see what the carb content is before you start to drink though.

Depending on what your overall calories are, you most likely would be able to have 1-2 light beers and be fine. Wine is similar to beer in this regard.

Most wines are going to contain too much sugar for it to be okay on a ketogenic diet. Even with this being the case though, you can have dry wine and be fine. Other alcoholic beverages that are acceptable on a ketogenic diet are whiskey, dry martinis, and plain vodka.

Again though, the main thing you want to be sure you do is to check and see how much sugar these beverages contain before you drink them. In the case of vodka for example, most of the time it's flavored, and the flavoring will add a bunch of sugar, which makes it bad for a ketogenic diet.

And even if you're consuming something such as a light beer, this doesn't mean that you have permission to go crazy.

Remember that you're still only allowed to eat 5% of your total calories from carbs.

Any alcohol you consume still has to fit within that. As long as you follow that rule and stick within the parameters of your macros, then you'll be good to go.

Can I Build Muscle and Burn Fat at the Same Time?

You might be interested in burning fat and building muscle. So is it possible to do both at the same time?

My answer to that would be that it depends. If someone already has a lot of muscle to begin with and is pretty lean, then it would be extremely hard for that individual to do both at the same time.

He would be much better off focusing on one goal at a time. On the other hand, if there's someone who's completely new to weightlifting and he has quite a bit of body fat to lose, then yes, it's certainly possible to burn fat and build muscle at the same time.

The thing is that you don't want to get caught up trying to chase two rabbit holes. It's better to focus on one goal at a time.

For example, if you have some extra fat to lose, but you also want to build some muscle, then focus solely on burning fat. The reality is that as a beginner, you can focus on burning fat and still build some muscle if you're lifting weights.

While it's technically possible to build muscle while you're in a caloric deficit, it's not optimal, which is why the advanced trainee would need to be in a caloric surplus in order to pack on some new size.

That's why it's best to focus on one goal at a time, and after achieving that goal, move onto the next goal and focus solely on that. For example, if someone currently weighs 200 pounds, he could lose the excess weight and get down to 170 pounds.

Then once he reaches that number, he could focus purely on building muscle. He could build 10 pounds of muscle to reach a bodyweight of 180. Think of any muscle you gain while you're trying to burn fat as a cool bonus and nothing more.

Don't go out of your way to try and make both happen at the same time because that could cause you to not achieve either goal.

How Can I Tell if I'm in the State of Ketosis?

The best way to know if you're in a state of ketosis or not is to test, test, test. There are a couple of different ways you can go about doing this.

The first method is to use urine test strips. Essentially you'll dip the test strip in a sample of your urine. Then after waiting roughly 15 seconds, a purplish color should start to appear on the strip.

A darker color of purple indicates a higher level of ketosis. A lighter shade of purple indicates lower levels of ketosis.

The key with the urine strips is to make sure that you have a consistent level of hydration when you take the test. You don't want to be dehydrated or super hydrated when you take the test.

Either of these two things can result in a false reading on the test. Instead, aim for your urine to have a slight yellow color to it and you should be good to go.

The other way you can test to see if you're in ketosis or not is to use a blood test. This is going to be a bit more expensive than the urine test strips, however, it's easier to get a more accurate and consistent reading.

You'll simply prick your finger and get an instant reading on the amount of ketones in your blood. Most of these test kits will come with a chart that'll show you if you currently have high or low levels of ketosis.

Finally, if you don't want to spend money on test kits, then there are some signs you can look out for to see if you're entering into a state of ketosis. These signs and symptoms are the same ones you'll experience if you get the keto flu.

These are things such as weakness, fatigue, headaches, nausea, and brain fog, among other things. However, if you're following the recommendations I outlined in the chapter on the keto flu, then it's possible that you might greatly lessen or even prevent the onset of the symptoms to begin with.

That's why using these symptoms to gauge if you're entering into a state of ketosis or not can be tricky. Not only that, but let's say you get into ketosis and then later on down the line you eat more carbs than you should have.

You're not sure if you ate too many carbs to kick you out of ketosis. The only way you'd be able to tell if you did get kicked out of ketosis is if you test for it.

Once you test for it, you can confirm whether or not you did indeed get kicked out of ketosis. After this, you can test along the way to know when you get back into ketosis.

What Are Some Examples of Things I Can Have on a Dirty Keto Diet that Aren't Allowed on a Standard Keto Diet?

On a normal ketogenic diet, everything you eat needs to be wholesome (i.e. natural) and organic when possible. On a dirty ketogenic diet, you don't have to follow that. You can essentially eat what you want as long as it contains a low amount of carbs, and you're still on track to hit your daily protein and fat macros.

This means that you can eat certain things such as processed foods, fast food, and drinks that contain artificial sweeteners. An example of this might be getting a bacon, egg, and cheese breakfast sandwich from a fast food restaurant.

You obviously wouldn't be able to eat the English muffin part of it, but everything else would be approved on a dirty ketogenic diet. However, on a strict or standard ketogenic diet, this breakfast item wouldn't be approved because of how it's been processed and prepared.

Another example would be something such as pork rinds. It's fine on a dirty keto diet, but because it's a processed food, it isn't approved on the standard keto diet.

So since this is a dirty keto diet, does that mean you can go crazy and eat whatever processed foods you want, whenever you want? Well, look at the next question for the answer to that...

How Should I Balance Eating Processed Foods with Clean Wholesome Foods?

Even though you technically could eat nothing but processed foods, that doesn't mean that you should. The reason for this is because you won't feel as good energy-wise if you eat nothing but junk food.

These foods items also contain a higher amount of calories in general than wholesome foods do. This is definitely something you'll want to think about because you're overall calories are going to be restricted since you're trying to lose weight.

Finally, wholesome foods such as vegetables are high in fiber, which is something that'll help you stay fuller for a longer period of time. You'll definitely want to take advantage of that when you're on a weight loss diet.

On the flip side, you don't want to eat clean foods all of the time either. This can make the diet plan hard to keep up with for the long haul. It could also make it more likely that you'll cheat on the diet, feel guilty, and then binge eat.

So there does need to be a proper balance between the two. The best way I've found to hit that balance is to eat clean wholesome foods 85% of the time. For the remaining 15% of the time, eat the processed foods that are allowed on the dirty ketogenic diet.

This allows you to enjoy certain food items you like from time to time, but it's not enough to make you feel sick from all of the junk food and potentially ruin the diet plan.

Remember that it's not what you eat 15% of the time that causes health problems—it's what you eat the majority of the time that can ruin your health. If you like eating pork rinds for example, and that helps to keep you moving forward, then by all means do it.

You just have to do so in the right amount. Eating an entire bag of pork rinds every single day would be too extreme, even for a dirty keto diet.

Having some from time to time is perfectly fine. As long as you strike a balance, you'll be good to go. And the best way to go about doing that is to eat natural foods 85% of the time and non-wholesome keto-approved foods the remaining 15% of the time.

Conclusion

You now have everything you need in order to be successful with this dirty keto diet plan. All that's left for you to do is execute on the plan.

There will certainly be some bumps in the road, but as long as you stay strong and persistent, you'll make it to your end destination. This diet plan will work as long as you stick to it.

If you give up and quit, then you won't be able to achieve your goal. Therefore, stick with it during good times and bad times. It'll be well worth it, so don't give up!

Did you enjoy reading this book? If so, please consider leaving a review. Even just a few words would help others decide if the book is right for them.

Best regards and thanks in advance—Thomas

Sources

(1) https://www.ncbi.nlm.nih.gov/pubmed/22825659

(2) https://www.ncbi.nlm.nih.gov/pubmed/14596707

(3)
https://www.ncbi.nlm.nih.gov/pmc/articles/PMC4434546/

Made in the USA
Middletown, DE
04 September 2019